Grappling Basics:
A New Twist on Conditioning

Brian Jones, M.S.

IronMind Enterprises, Inc.
Nevada City, California

All rights reserved. No part of this book may be reproduced or transmitted in any form or by any means without written permission except in the case of brief quotations embodied in articles or reviews. For further information, please contact the publisher.

Grappling Basics: A New Twist on Conditioning

©2008 IronMind Enterprises, Inc.

Cataloging in Publication Data
Jones, Brian—
Grappling basics: a new twist on conditioning
1. Fitness and health   2. Martial arts   I. Title
Library of Congress Control Number: 2008939976
ISBN-13: 978-0-926888-79-1
Book cover and design by Tony Agpoon, Sausalito, California

Photo credits: Brian Jones, Tracy Wright, James Butler, Chad Talkington, and Michael Seals

Models: Brian Jones, Greg Holden, James Liau, Ryan Jones, James Butler, and Tony Mancuso

Published in the United States of America
IronMind Enterprises, Inc., P.O. Box 1228, Nevada City, CA 95959

Printed in the USA. First Edition
10 9 8 7 6 5 4 3 2

With love to Tracy.

Table of Contents

Introduction   2

Chapter 1 – Stances, Footwork, and Movement   6
     Stances   6
     Footwork   8
     Movement   10

Chapter 2 – Clinch Work and Takedowns   20
     Clinch Work (Tie-ups)   20
     Takedowns   26

Chapter 3 – Ground Positioning and Pins   38
     Overview of Positions   38
     Mount   41
     Cross Side   46
     Scarf Hold   49
     Back Mount   52
     Guard   54

Chapter 4 – Submission   64
     Joint Locks   65
     Chokes   70

Chapter 5 – Exercises and Drills   74
     Bodyweight Grappling Drills   74
     Partner Resistance Training   89

Chapter 6 – Workout and Program Design   102
     Short Cycle Workouts   104
     Dynamic Workouts   106
     Integration Workouts   106
     Combative Drilling and Conditioning   108

Index   110

About the Author

Brian Jones has an M.S. in exercise physiology and is a doctoral candidate at the University of Kentucky. He has been involved in strength and conditioning for many years and has trained athletes in a variety of sports from the high school to professional level. A judo and Brazilian jiu-jitsu instructor, Brian is especially interested in strength and conditioning as it applies to competitive fighters. Brian is the author of the popular *Complete Sandbag Training Course,* which has made sandbag training a staple in many strength and conditioning programs, and *The Conditioning Handbook: Getting in Top Shape,* an A-to-Z guide to endurance training.

Acknowledgements

I would like to thank the staff of Four Seasons Martial Arts for the use of their facility and everyone who was involved in any way in the production of this book. Special thanks to Tracy Wright for her help and support.

Other IronMind Enterprises, Inc. Publications

SUPER SQUATS: How to Gain 30 Pounds of Muscle in 6 Weeks by Randall J. Strossen, Ph.D.

The Complete Keys to Progress by John McCallum, edited by Randall J. Strossen, Ph.D.

Mastery of Hand Strength, Revised Edition by John Brookfield

IronMind: Stronger Minds, Stronger Bodies by Randall J. Strossen, Ph.D.

MILO: A Journal for Serious Strength Athletes, Randall J. Strossen, Ph.D., Publisher and Editor-in-chief

Powerlifting Basics, Texas-style: The Adventures of Lope Delk by Paul Kelso

Of Stones and Strength by Steve Jeck and Peter Martin

Sons of Samson, Volume 2 by David Webster

Rock Iron Steel: The Book of Strength by Steve Justa

Paul Anderson: The Mightiest Minister by Randall J. Strossen, Ph.D.

Louis Cyr: Amazing Canadian by Ben Weider, C.M.

Training with Cables for Strength by John Brookfield

The Grip Master's Manual by John Brookfield

Captains of Crush® Grippers: What They Are and How to Close Them by Randall J. Strossen, Ph.D., J. B. Kinney, and Nathan Holle

Winning Ways: How to Succeed In the Gym and Out by Randall J. Strossen, Ph.D.

The Complete Sandbag Training Course by Brian Jones, M.S.

Bodyweight Exercises for Extraordinary Strength by Brad Johnson

The Conditioning Handbook: Getting in Top Shape by Brian Jones, M.S.

To order additional copies of *Grappling Basics: A New Twist on Conditioning* or for a catalog of IronMind Enterprises, Inc. publications and products, please contact:

IronMind Enterprises, Inc.
P.O. Box 1228
Nevada City, CA 95959 USA
tel: 530-272-3579
fax: 530-272-3095
website: www.ironmind.com
e-mail: sales@ironmind.com

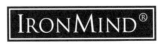

Stronger Minds, Stronger Bodies™

Introduction

Grappling, or combat sport involving grabbing, throwing, and submission holds, is just as popular today as it has been throughout history. Its longevity and its timelessness are for good reason, as grappling combines self-defense skills with strength, endurance, power, and flexibility to form one of the most complete modes of physical training available.

Grappling is one of the oldest and most universal of all human activities. It has existed in the context of war, sport, or ritual since the beginning of recorded history. *The Epic of Gilgamesh* (2750–2500 BC), one of the earliest known literary works, describes a wrestling match between Gilgamesh and a wild brute named Enkidu sent by the gods to challenge him. Ancient Egyptian scrolls and hieroglyphics, dating as far back as 2300 BC, depict wrestlers performing many of the techniques common in modern grappling. Perhaps better known to most readers are the ancient Greeks, who included wrestling and a style of mixed martial arts called *pankration* in their Olympics.

Every known culture the world over has its indigenous form of wrestling. From the frozen north of Iceland comes *glima*, a traditional style that was once the sport of Vikings. Tribes in the parched lands of sub-Saharan Africa still participate in a kind of wrestling descended from the ancient Nubians. Popular grappling styles, such as freestyle, Greco-Roman, sambo, judo, and jiu-jitsu, are modern sportive versions derived from more traditional arts.

The universal appeal of grappling is easy to understand. It requires no equipment or facilities and is thus accessible to all people, regardless of wealth or social status. The outcome of a grappling match is based entirely on skill, strength, and conditioning unmediated by technology or chance. There are no teammates on whom one can rely for success, or blame for failure. Other than minor changes in technique and training methods, no differences exist between the modern grappling athlete and his ancient counterpart. Grappling is the distilled essence of individualized raw human competition.

Grappling is the distilled essence of individualized raw human competition.

Unlike other more specialized sports, grappling demands and develops all aspects of human fitness. It requires balance, agility, and the ability to control one's own bodyweight in space. Resisting an opponent involves high-intensity loads and sharp, powerful movements. The nearly inexhaustible range of techniques available to the grappler means that almost every human motion possible is used to some degree. Pushing, pulling, squatting, lifting, and twisting through different and constantly changing ranges of motion are all present during workouts. In addition, the demands on muscular and cardiovascular endurance are dramatic, as any new trainee will immediately learn.

It is for these reasons that grappling has always enjoyed a prominent place in physical culture. Almost without exception, the European and American strongmen throughout the nineteenth and early twentieth centuries used grappling as part of their training. Some were wrestlers first and strongmen second, in the cases of Frank Gotch, Martin "Farmer" Burns, and George "The Russian Lion" Hackenschmidt. Other iron game legends, like the great Arthur Saxon and Earle Leiderman, trained in wrestling as well as with weights and performed challenge matches along with feats of strength for their audiences. For many, the physical domination of a resisting opponent was the truest test of "functional" strength.

For many, the physical domination of a resisting opponent was the truest test of "functional" strength.

The trend in the modern age is one of specialization rather than generalization. Sports and fitness activities have become increasingly more focused and refined. In some ways specialization is positive and necessary: more intense focus encourages exceptional development in a given area. World records have fallen continually as coaches, athletes, and scientists have pushed the envelope of human performance. Techniques and training methods approach ever more closely the boundaries of what is physiologically and psychologically possible; as training methods improve, we can come closer to the absolute limits of human performance.

However, in this maddening race, something has been left behind. No matter how often two strong men might compete by adding weight in turns to the bar, the question presents itself, what if there were no bar? Who would win then?

The purpose of *Grappling Basics: A New Twist on Conditioning* is to reintroduce grappling into physical culture. Physical culture was and is intended to be a system of holistic training, not merely bodybuilding. For the physical culturist, training encompasses form, function, health, and will. The greatest of the old-time strongmen recognized and used grappling training as a valuable supplement to their lifting and competed in grappling matches to demonstrate their physical prowess. Hopefully, this book will stimulate an interest in grappling as an adjunct method of physical training in those lifters who might otherwise not have tried it. *Grappling Basics: A New Twist on Conditioning* is designed to give the non-grappler a foundational level of skill for further practice. By practicing the techniques and incorporating the exercises into their routines, new trainees can obtain levels of functional strength otherwise not possible.

For those with grappling experience, *Grappling Basics: A New Twist on Conditioning* is an excellent resource for conditioning programs using grappling-specific exercises. Even the experienced grappler should come away with some useful ideas on how to create effective sport-specific conditioning programs.

Chapter 1 introduces the foundations of grappling: stances, footwork, and movement. Mastering this material is key for the techniques that follow. In Chapter 2, the basics of the takedown are covered. It includes how to properly tie up with an opponent from the standing position and take him to the mat. Once the match goes to the ground, the pinning and control techniques of Chapter 3 are vital for dominating the opponent. Chapter 4 details several submission holds that can be applied to force your opponent to give up. The latter section of the book, Chapters 5 and 6, describes many different grappling-based exercises and drills—useful for increasing both skill and fitness—and how to incorporate them into your training. The best approach for the reader is to move through the book sequentially in order not to miss any important steps.

Author's Note: Throughout this book I use the masculine pronouns he, his, and him as a convention of language. Women and men alike can and should incorporate grappling training into their programs.

Grappling Basics: A New Twist on Conditioning

Chapter 1

Stances, Footwork, and Movement

Stances, footwork, and movement form the basis for all further grappling skills. Proficiency with these techniques and principles is a prerequisite for the material later in the book. Faulty stances, poor footwork, and awkward movement will place you at a disadvantage during offense and defense. Practice these skills extensively and often. Consider using some of them for warm-ups during every training session. For solo trainees who don't intend to compete, these exercises are challenging, interesting and effective for building functional strength and athletic ability.

Stances

While there are many variations of the basic grappling stance, all of them have three things in common:
- First, they place you in a balanced position. Without balance you will be unable to attack or defend properly.
- Second, they allow you to move quickly and easily in any direction. Grappling is a fast-paced, dynamic sport, and you must be able to initiate your attacks or defensive moves without hesitation.
- Third, they provide protection. Proper placement of your arms, legs, and head makes it difficult for your opponent to take you down.

With these ideas in mind, take a look at the basic staggered stance shown in Figure 1.

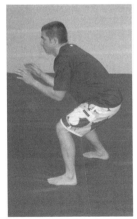

Figure 1.
Basic staggered stance, left side.

The key technical points are:

- **Head** – Your head is up, shoulders slightly elevated, and eyes forward. This position makes it difficult for your opponent to control your head with a headlock or guillotine choke, or to force you to the mat with a snap-down.

- **Arms** – Your arms are in what is called a "forklift" position, with your elbows tight to your sides and forearms perpendicular to your body. This position prevents your opponent from controlling your body with the various tie-up moves discussed in Chapter 2 and makes it easier to defend against double- or single-leg takedowns.

- **Trunk** – Your body is bent slightly forward at the waist, making it more difficult for your opponent to get under you and execute a takedown.

- **Knees** – Your knees are bent slightly. Maintaining a crouch makes it easier to move and change your level to attack and defend.

- **Feet** – Your weight is on the balls of your feet. It is essential that you stay off your heels when grappling. Getting caught on your heels roots you to the ground and limits your mobility.

Notice the three stances shown in Figures 2 through 4.

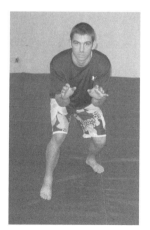

Figure 2.
Staggered stance,
right foot lead.

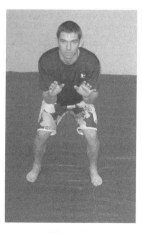

Figure 3.
Square stance.

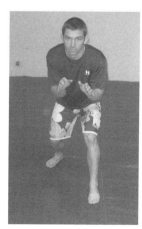

Figure 4.
Staggered stance,
left foot lead.

Grappling Basics: A New Twist on Conditioning

You can lead with either foot in a staggered stance. The middle stance is referred to as a square stance and is a transitional position used primarily for circling your opponent. Although it is common to switch stances during grappling, you should specialize in either the left- or right-lead stance. Try both and focus on the one that feels more comfortable. Your technical skill will improve more quickly if you train mostly on one side. If your primary reason for grappling is strength and conditioning work, feel free to work both sides evenly on all the drills.

Footwork

Grappling is a fast-paced, dynamic sport so the right stance means nothing if you can't move properly. Proper footwork keeps you balanced and ready to attack or defend. You should initiate and finish all movement in a solid stance. Footwork is one of those foundational skills to which beginners and advanced athletes should devote ample time. After you develop a basic proficiency, continue to monitor your technique as you work to develop more advanced skills. New skills require a lot of attention and can sometimes disrupt more fundamental ones.

<u>Front and back – linear</u>
To move straight forward from the basic left-lead staggered stance, push off your back foot and step forward with your lead leg. Bring your back foot up and regain your stance. To move backward press off the lead foot, step back with your rear leg, and then step your lead foot back to regain your stance. Keep your upper-body position constant while stepping. Avoid the common mistake of switching leads on each step. Always step first with the front leg when moving forward and with the rear leg when moving backward.

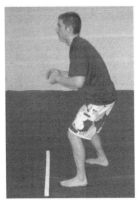
Figure 5.
Step forward, basic left-lead stance.

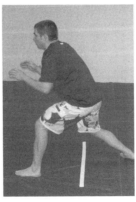
Figure 6.
Step forward, push off rear leg.

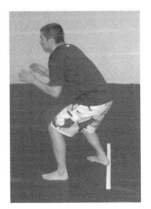
Figure 7.
Step forward, return to basic staggered stance.

Left and right – lateral
When stepping left from a left-lead staggered stance, step your lead (left) foot first; then move your rear leg over to regain your stance. Step right by moving the rear (right) leg first and moving your lead (left) leg over to regain your stance. Conversely, when stepping right from a right-lead staggered stance, step your lead (right) foot first; then move your rear (left) leg over to regain your stance. Step left by moving the rear (left) leg first and moving your lead (right) leg over to regain your stance.

Just as with the front and back motion, maintain your upper-body position while moving. A common mistake is to move the wrong foot first, resulting in a crossover step. If your opponent attacks while your feet are crossed, it will be very difficult to defend.

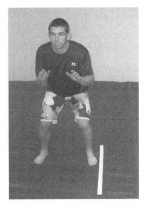
Figure 8.
Lateral step, start.

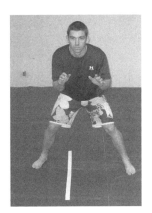
Figure 9.
Lateral step, lead leg.

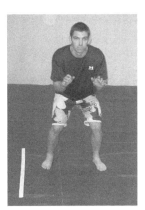
Figure 10.
Lateral step, finish.

Circling
The circling motion is less a step and more a sliding shuffle. During circling you will make a transition from a staggered stance to the square stance described above. Move left by stepping with your left foot first and then sliding your right foot up; move right by stepping with your right foot first and then moving your left. The key to a stable circling stance is to keep low. Avoid the common mistake of bouncing up and down with each step as this will put you in a weak defensive position if your opponent attacks.

Movement

Level change

Changing your level, or the height of your stance, is a key move in both offense and defense. Most takedowns involve lowering your level so that you can get under your opponent's defenses. Conversely, stopping the takedown requires that you change your level when your opponent does so that he cannot get under you. A quick level change can also be used to fake out your opponent and help set up your techniques.

The motion is almost exclusively in the legs. Keep your lower back, arms, and head in the same position and bend your knees to change levels. The drops can be shallow (only 6 or 8 inches) or deep (touching your knee to the mat); regardless of the depth, you must change levels quickly and then explode back up.

Sprawling
The sprawl is technically a defensive move against a single- or double-leg shot, but I include it here because it is so fundamental. Sprawling is an extreme form of level change used when your opponent attempts to grab your legs. The goal is to get your hips down and throw your legs back as far as possible.

Look at the sequence shown in Figures 11 and 12.

Figure 11 shows the grappler in a proper staggered stance. From here, he throws his legs backward and drops quickly to the mat (Figure 12). Since he started in a left-

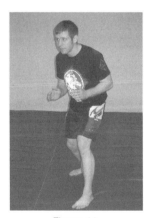

Figure 11.
Sprawling, start.

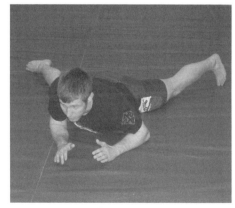

Figure 12.
Sprawling, finish.

lead stance, he will twist his hips to the right. This movement is essential to help break any grip the opponent might have on your lead leg. The key to sprawling is to drop quickly and drive your hips into the mat. Sprawling is vital but not necessarily comfortable, and it must be done on a mat for safety.

Falling

To practice takedowns safely you must learn how to fall. Grappling arts such as judo, where throwing is a major part of competition, spend a great deal of time working on breakfalls. Arts like Brazilian jiu-jitsu, which spend most of the time grappling on the mat, do not emphasize falling as much. Every grappler should have a basic proficiency with falling techniques for two reasons. First is the safety aspect that we have already mentioned: sprains, breaks, dislocations, and concussions can occur easily with poor technique. The second, and little discussed, reason for learning to fall is that it will improve the quality of your practice. If you are not comfortable landing, it will be almost impossible to relax and let your training partner throw you. You will stiffen up and unconsciously defend every rep.

Back falls
Start the back fall in a standing position with your arms crossed on your chest. Squat down and roll onto your back. Keep your chin tucked to your chest, exhale on impact, and slap the mat with your forearms and hands. Slapping the mat will help you build awareness of where your hands are on impact, and it will teach you to land with maximal surface area. Landing hands- or elbows-first can seriously damage the shoulder, elbow, or wrist joints. Allow your body to roll backward slightly so that your legs can come up.

Side falls
The side fall to the left begins with the right leg forward. Hold your left arm up to your chest. Swing your left leg and left arm across your body as shown in Figure 14 and sit down on your left side. Slap the mat with your left arm, as shown in Figure 15. For a right side fall, begin with the left leg forward and do the same movements on the opposite side. Just as in the back fall, be sure to exhale, tuck your chin, and allow your body to roll slightly backward.

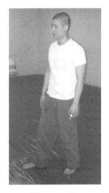
Figure 13.
Side fall, start.

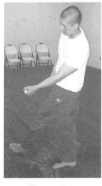
Figure 14.
Side fall, leg swing.

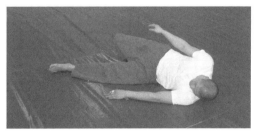
Figure 15.
Side fall, finish.

Front falls

The front fall starts from a standing position, with your arms out in front of you or crossed on your chest. Squat and kick your legs back. Tuck your arms in and land on your palms and forearms. Keep your head up to prevent it from hitting the floor, and exhale on impact.

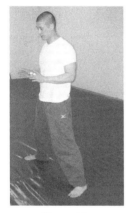
Figure 16.
Front fall, start.

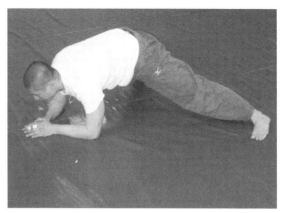
Figure 17.
Front fall, finish.

Spin-outs

Some wrestling styles award a higher score for throwing an opponent directly on his back (judo, sambo, freestyle, and Greco wrestling), while others score all takedowns in the same way regardless of landing position (Brazilian jiu-jitsu and submission wrestling). In the latter cases, you want to hit the mat on your back if possible so that you can get into the guard position rather than having the opponent get on your back.

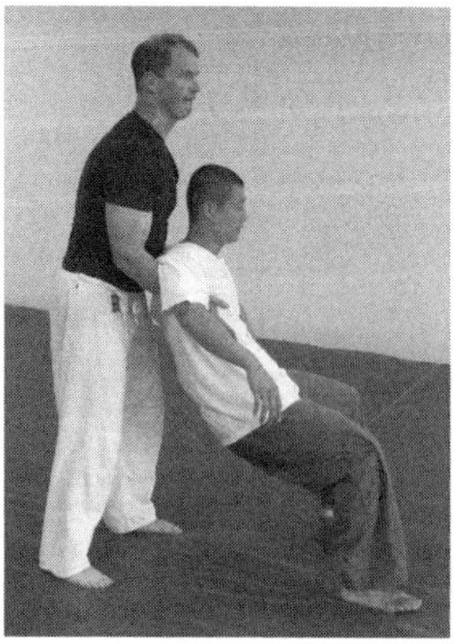

Spin-out drills teach you to rotate your body in the air so that you can minimize the advantage to your opponent if you are taken down. They can be done back to front or front to back. If you are training to compete in a particular grappling style, you may want to stick to the drill that most applies to those rules. Otherwise, use both methods to develop greater body control.

Figure 18.
Partner supported spin-out, eyes closed.

The back-to-front drill starts with a back fall. As you start to fall, twist your body in mid-air and land in the front fall position. Learn to twist to both sides. You can do this drill from a squatting or standing position, or by leaping backward, depending on your skill and comfort level. Another advanced variation involves closing your eyes and having a partner support you, as in Figure 18. Have him release you without warning to challenge your reflexes.

Progression

Falling from a standing position can be intimidating at first. A useful progression for beginners learning these falls is to start first from a squatting position, as shown in Figures 19 through 21.

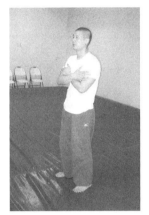
Figure 19.
Back fall, start.

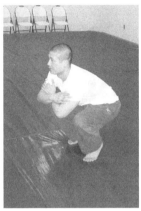
Figure 20.
Back fall, squatting position.

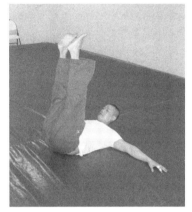
Figure 21.
Back fall from squat position, finish.

This sequence reduces the impact and helps to build confidence. As your skill improves, gradually increase the height of your squat until you are standing.

Although the impact can be rather severe, more advanced trainees should practice occasional reps by leaping into the falls. This movement more closely simulates absorbing a hard takedown in sparring. Before attempting these jumping falls, be sure you have mastered the basics and are using a wrestling or judo mat.

Rolling and tumbling

All grapplers should become proficient at basic rolling and tumbling techniques, as they teach safe falling, agility, and kinesthetic awareness. You do not have to become as skilled as a gymnast to benefit from these movements. Work into these movements slowly to avoid injury. At first they will make you extremely dizzy, but with practice your body will adjust.

Forward somersault roll

Starting from a standing position, squat down and put both hands on the mat. Tuck your chin to your chest and your knees to your body, and roll forward. Stay in the tucked position throughout the roll. You should end up in the starting position.

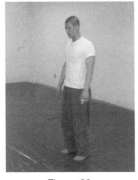
Figure 22.
Forward somersault roll, start.

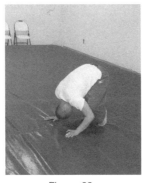
Figure 23.
Forward somersault roll, tuck.

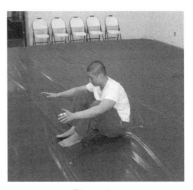
Figure 24.
Forward somersault roll, finish.

Backward somersault roll

From a standing position, squat down, tuck your knees and head, and roll backward. Use your abdominal muscles to help generate the necessary momentum. This exercise is usually more difficult to learn than the forward roll as you will have a tendency to become untucked. Again, you should end up in the starting position.

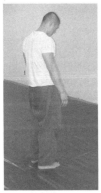
Figure 25.
Backward somersault roll, start.

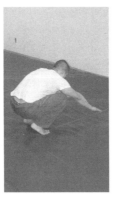
Figure 26.
Backward somersault roll, squat.

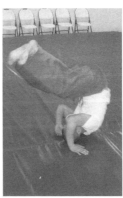
Figure 27.
Backward somersault roll, push over.

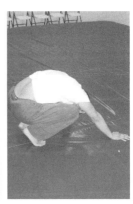
Figure 28.
Backward somersault roll, finish.

Forward shoulder roll

Shoulder rolls differ from somersault rolls in that you are rolling diagonally across your shoulder and back, rather than straight over your head. Start standing with your left leg forward. Tuck your chin; reach across your body with your left arm toward your right leg. Make gradual contact with the mat, starting with the blade of your left hand; roll across your arm and left shoulder. You can continue the roll all the way to a standing position or stop in the side fall position (Figure 32).

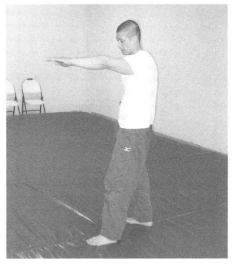

Figure 29.
Forward shoulder roll, start.

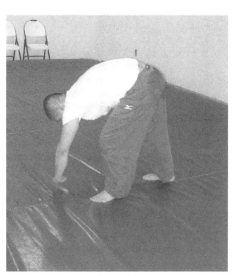

Figure 30.
Forward shoulder roll, reach.

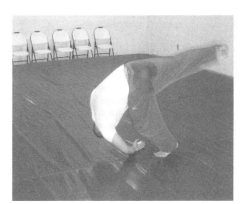

Figure 31.
Forward shoulder roll, arm and shoulder.

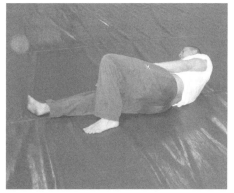

Figure 32.
Forward shoulder roll, finish.

Grappling Basics: A New Twist on Conditioning | **15**

Backward shoulder roll

From a standing position, squat down and stretch both arms out at your sides. Roll backward by throwing your legs over and to one side, and rolling over your shoulder rather than straight over your neck. Come up into a kneeling position. Many people have difficulty at first with this movement. If you can't prevent rolling over your neck, practice throwing your legs up and over your head to one side and then the other.

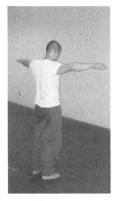
Figure 33. Backward shoulder roll, start.

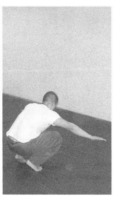
Figure 34. Backward shoulder roll, squat.

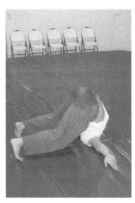
Figure 35. Backward shoulder roll, leg throw.

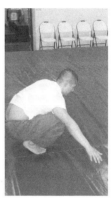
Figure 36. Backward shoulder roll, finish.

Cartwheels and roundoffs

Cartwheels and roundoffs are two fundamental tumbling skills that all grapplers should develop. They build confidence, agility, and the ability to move your body through space when throwing or being thrown.

The key technical point on the cartwheel is to keep your arms and body straight throughout the movement so that you roll like a wheel. Try to get full extension on your arms and legs and keep your legs spread, as shown in Figure 38. Your chest should remain vertical throughout. Common errors are doing the movement with your chest facing the floor or allowing your chest to twist. Once you have developed some proficiency with the cartwheel, move on to the roundoff.

A roundoff starts the same way as the cartwheel. However, once you have reached the fully-extended overhead position, twist your body using the strength of your core muscles so that you land on your feet facing in the opposite direction, as shown in Figure 40. Focus on twisting from the core and bringing your feet to the mat as quickly as possible.

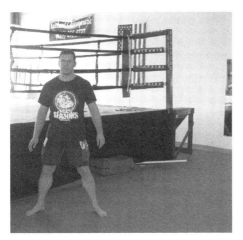
Figure 37.
Cartwheel and roundoff, starting position.

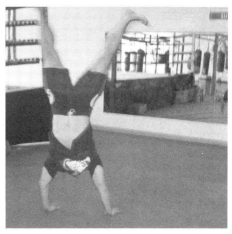
Figure 38.
Cartwheel and roundoff, full extension.

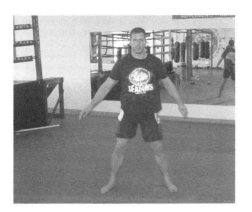
Figure 39.
Cartwheel, finish.

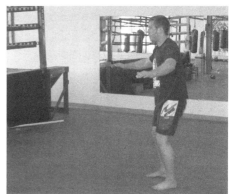
Figure 40.
Roundoff, finish.

Crawls

Crawling drills improve mat mobility and build endurance throughout the body, particularly in the arms and shoulders. There are several different methods of crawling and each variation will provide you with a different type of workout. In addition to building skill, these drills make good warm-ups or complete workouts.

Bear crawl

Crawl on all fours with only your hands and feet touching the mat. Stay low and keep your hips down to increase the stress on your arms. From the basic position shown in Figure 41, you can move in any direction.

Crab crawl

Start on all fours with your chest facing up, and move without allowing your body to touch the mat. As in the bear crawl, this drill should be practiced moving in all directions. Crab crawls place quite a bit of stress on the shoulders, elbows, and wrists. Use caution if you have any injuries in these areas.

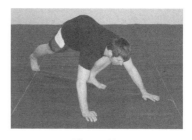

Figure 41.
Bear crawl.

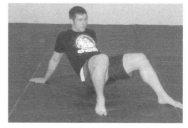

Figure 42.
Crab crawl.

Standing up

Standing up properly is one of the key movement skills in grappling. Start on the ground in the position shown in Figure 43. Place your weight on your right hand and your left foot and lift your hip off the mat. Swivel your right leg back under your body and stand up into a solid wrestling stance. Practice this technique on both sides.

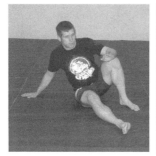 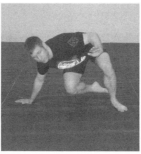 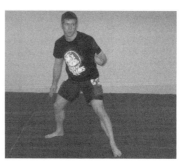

Figure 43.
Standing up, start.

Figure 44.
Standing up, hip lift, leg swivel.

Figure 45.
Standing up, finish.

Grappling Basics: A New Twist on Conditioning | **19**

Chapter 2: Clinch Work and Takedowns

This chapter covers the fundamentals of stand-up grappling. It shows how to tie up, or grip, your opponent when both of you are standing, and how to work takedowns, both attack and defense, from this standing tied-up range—often termed the "clinch." Around fifty percent of the grappling game takes place on the feet, and if you don't know how to stop a takedown, you will be at an extreme disadvantage. The clinch is also very important for self-defense as most fights tend to quickly end up in this range.

Clinch Work (Tie-ups)

Wrist control

As you move close to your opponent, one of the first opportunities you will have to make contact and control him will be by grabbing his wrist. Always grab the wrist of the arm closest to you. If you reach for the far wrist, you risk overextending yourself and getting out of position. Grip, using either an overhand or underhand position, and hold tightly so that your opponent cannot pull his hand away. If your opponent does not fight

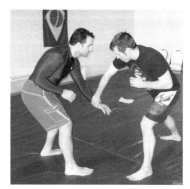
Figure 46.
Wrist control, grab nearest wrist.

against the grip, use it to control the arm and set up further tie-ups. If he pulls away violently, release the grip and execute a takedown or body-lock while he is out of position (these are described later in this chapter).

From a defensive standpoint, prevent the opponent from grabbing your wrist by maintaining a proper wrestling stance, with your elbows in. If he grabs your wrist, bring your other hand over to grab his wrist and remove his hand. If he has an overhand grip, pull his wrist in while you pull your arm away (Figures 47 and 48).

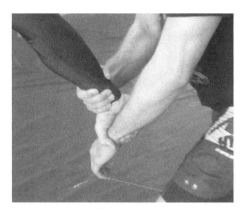
Figure 47.
Overhand grip release, start.

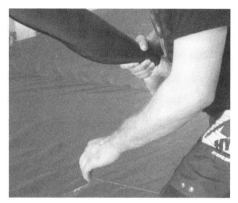
Figure 48.
Overhand grip release, finish.

To remove an underhand grip, push his wrist out while you pull your arm away (Figures 49 and 50). Always use short, quick motions to remove the grip, and stay in a proper stance while performing them.

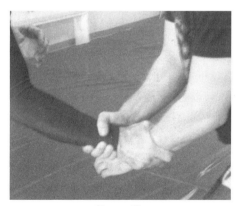
Figure 49.
Underhand grip release, start.

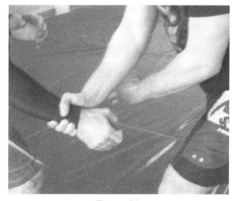
Figure 50.
Underhand grip release, finish.

Practice these techniques using a drill called hand fighting. Face off with your partner and work to establish and maintain wrist control. Your partner will do the same. The drill will be a continuous series of grabs, releases, and regrabs.

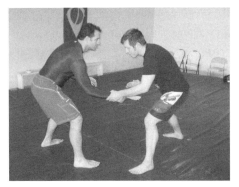
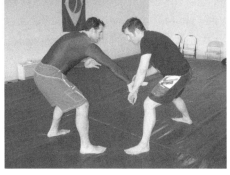
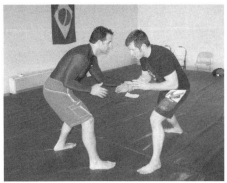
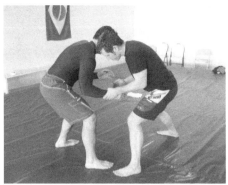

Figures 51–54.
Hand fighting, grabs and releases.

Head and wrist tie-up

Learning how to tie up with your opponent and control him is essential for successful takedowns and takedown defense. The two tie-ups and grips illustrated are the most common and most effective. Grab the opponent's right wrist with your left hand in an underhand grip and bring his head into your right shoulder with your right hand behind his neck (Figure 55). Do the same move on the other side with opposite hands (Figure 56). When you and your partner tie up with one another, you should always get into one of these positions rather than just grabbing blindly.

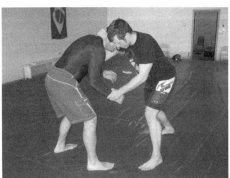
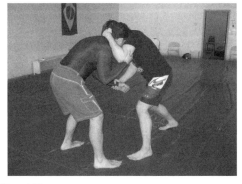

Figures 55 and 56.
Head and wrist control.

Over-and-under position

The over-and-under position is one of the most common tie-ups in grappling. As you come to grips with your opponent, your right arm will be under your opponent's left arm, and your left arm will be on the outside of his right arm gripping at his elbow. You will be pressing forward slightly to maintain close chest contact. This is considered a neutral position in that neither you nor your opponent has a decided advantage of control. Practice this position on both sides and learn to move around the mat freely and with balance, while putting pressure on your opponent. You will use this position to set up several different moves.

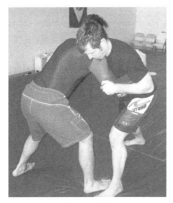
Figure 57.
Over-and-under position, side one.

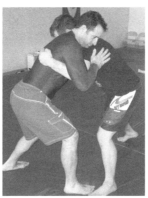
Figure 58.
Over-and-under position, side two.

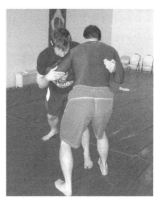
Figure 59.
Over-and-under position, front view.

Front body-lock and pummeling

To gain more control over your opponent, you can move from the over-and-under position into the front body-lock shown in Figure 60. In the body-lock, you have both arms under your opponent's arms and your hips dropped lower to get under him. Your hands will be locked around his lower back as shown.

Getting from the over-and-under position to the front body-lock is accomplished by swimming your left arm inside the opponent's right arm and locking your hands behind your opponent's lower back. Drop your level and step into your opponent to get under him.

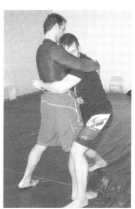
Figure 60.
Front body-lock.

Grappling Basics: A New Twist on Conditioning | **23**

The swimming movement of the arms is practiced cooperatively in a drill known as pummeling. Swim your left arm under your opponent's right arm as he does the same thing to you. Move your head to the other side so that you are in the over-and-under position again on the opposite side. Repeat this drill, going from side to side. Maintain chest contact throughout. Pummeling should be done slowly and cooperatively at first; you can gradually build up speed and add resistance when you improve.

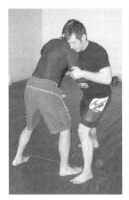

Figure 61.
Pummeling, start.

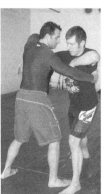

Figures 62 and 63.
Pummeling, swim arms.

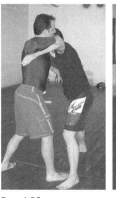

Figure 64.
Pummeling, finish on other side.

Head and elbow

Another common tie-up position is the head and elbow. Grab the back of your opponent's neck with your right hand and grab his right arm at the elbow with your left hand. Pull your right elbow down so that it is against your opponent's chest and keep a downward pull on his head. Your left hand grips at the crook of the opponent's elbow. Drill this position by moving around the mat. Pull your opponent forward and down as you move to help break his balance. Your opponent will be doing the same to you, so be sure to keep your feet under you as you move. When he pulls you in, walk forward rather than allowing your upper body to get far ahead of your lower body, as shown in Figure 65. This is a weak, off-balance position that makes it easy for your opponent to score a takedown on you.

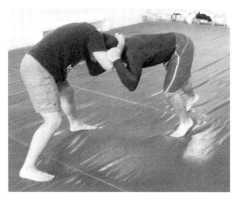

Figure 65.
Head and elbow, off-balance position.

Two-on-one (Russian)

The two-on-one tie-up (also called the Russian) is used to set up a number of takedowns. Reach out and grab your opponent's right wrist with your right hand. Simultaneously pull him forward as you step forward and toward his right side. Bring your left arm up under his right biceps and hug his arm tightly to your body. Apply pressure to his arm with your left shoulder. Typically, the opponent will attempt to pull his arm back in, so be sure to hold tightly. You will also have to circle to your right to prevent your opponent from circling back in to you.

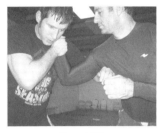

Figure 66.
Two-on-one, wrist grab, close-up view.

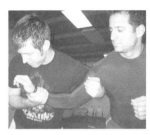

Figure 67.
Two-on-one, arm hug.

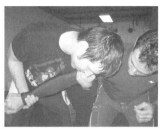

Figure 68.
Two-on-one, shoulder pressure.

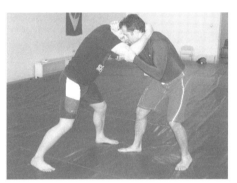

Figure 69.
Two-on-one, start, full view.

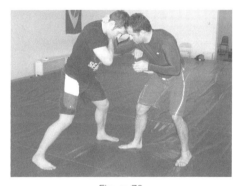

Figure 70.
Two-on-one, wrist grab.

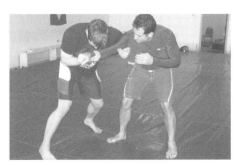

Figure 71.
Two-on-one, step and arm hug.

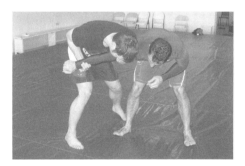

Figure 72.
Two-on-one, shoulder pressure.

Takedowns

Penetration step

The penetration step, also known as a shot, is a key component of several different common takedowns, including the single- and double-leg. Before moving on to the actual takedowns, it is important to become proficient with this movement. Begin in a proper wrestling stance. Drop your level and take a deep step forward by driving off your back foot. Allow your front knee to push forward over your front foot and touch down on the mat. Next, step forward by dragging your rear foot along the mat and to the front. Keep your chest and head up and elbows tucked at your sides throughout the motion. Practice the penetration step by "walking" along the mat until you can perform it rapidly and fluidly. Here is a list of the most common technical errors:

- Looking down – Keep your head up and chest forward. You should be looking straight ahead rather than at the ground.
- Bending at the waist – Drop your level by bending your knees. If you bend too far forward at the waist, you will be off-balance and out of position.
- Not dropping the front knee – Remember that this is not a lunge step as you might do in the weightroom. Your front knee must push forward over your front toe and continue all the way down to the mat.

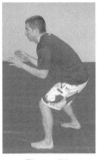
Figure 73.
Penetration step,
start.

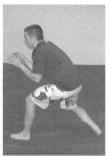
Figure 74.
Penetration step,
level drop.

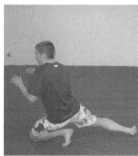
Figure 75.
Penetration step,
knee down.

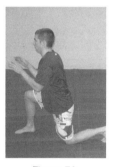
Figure 76.
Penetration step,
rear leg forward.

Double-leg takedown

Broadly defined, the double-leg takedown involves executing a penetration step as described above, and then taking your opponent to the mat by grabbing both of his legs. Although the penetration step is used as an entry, there are a number of different ways to finish. In this book we cover three of the most common and effective finishes.

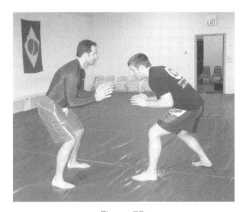
Figure 77.
Double-leg takedown, start.

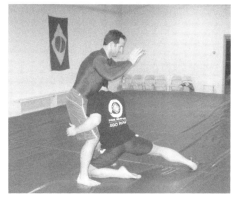
Figure 78.
Double-leg takedown, penetration step and leg grab.

<u>Drive-through</u>

If the opponent does not move his legs and hips backward into a defensive sprawl, you will finish by continuing the forward momentum and driving straight through him. As you hit the penetration step, use your hands to pull or chop at the back of the opponent's knees as you step forward with your back leg. Pulling the backs of his knees toward you will cause the opponent to collapse backward.

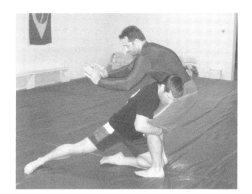
Figure 79.
Drive-through double-leg takedown, pull at knees.

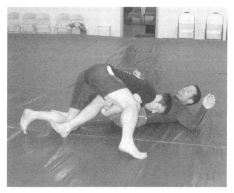
Figure 80.
Drive-through double-leg takedown, finish.

The most common technical error in this finish is losing forward momentum. Keep stepping forward using the penetration step with one-hundred-percent commitment.

Grappling Basics: A New Twist on Conditioning | **27**

Step behind trip

Sometimes it can be difficult to finish the drive-through if your partner keeps moving backward to defend the throw. To prevent this delay tactic, take another big forward penetration step after the first one and try to get your right leg behind your opponent's leg as shown in Figure 82. Once hooked behind, continue to drive forward. Your opponent will not be able to step back, and the pressure on the front of his knee will force him to fall.

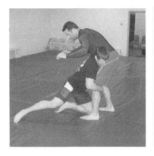
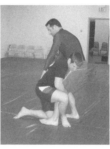
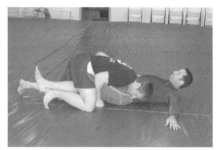

Figure 81.
Step behind trip, start.

Figure 82.
Step behind trip, leg hook.

Figure 83.
Step behind trip, finish.

As in the drive-through, the most common error in the step behind trip is losing forward momentum. You must keep driving and take a large, exaggerated step behind the opponent's leg in order to finish.

Turn the corner

An experienced opponent, or even someone with good balance, will instinctively throw his hips back to get his legs out of the way in a movement known as a sprawl (see page 10). This defensive technique will often prevent you from driving forward to finish the throw. Rather than continuing your forward drive, take a large outside step with the right leg and turn in a circle to your right. Push the opponent toward the left with your head and lift up on his left leg to turn him to the mat.

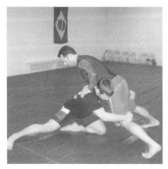
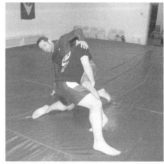
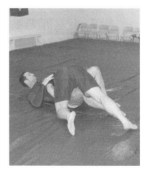

Figure 84.
Turn the corner, sprawl attempt.

Figure 85.
Turn the corner, outside step and circle.

Figure 86.
Turn the corner, opponent to mat.

One common error is taking too shallow a circle step. Step in deep, and then turn the corner hard. Another problem is not using the head to push the opponent. Always step to the side that your head is on; otherwise, you will crank your own neck when you attempt this finish. As you turn the circle, push hard into the opponent's side with your head.

Single-leg takedown

The single-leg takedown involves using a quick level change to capture one of the opponent's legs. Once you control the leg, there are a number of different finishes or methods for getting the opponent to the mat. Always attack the forward leg when your opponent is in a staggered stance because it can be grabbed faster and it is more difficult for your opponent to defend. To get the opponent's leg, drop your level quickly and grab with both arms and pinch his leg between your legs as shown in Figure 87. Keep your body tight against his thigh and your head in by his stomach.

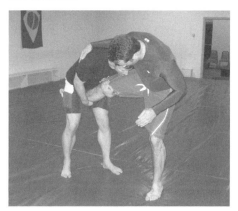
Figure 87.
Single-leg takedown.

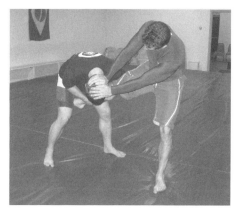
Figure 88.
Single-leg takedown, head too far away.

A common error is not holding on tightly enough to the captured leg. A loose grip will allow your opponent to free his leg and escape. Another problem is keeping your head too far away from the opponent's leg, as shown in Figure 88. If you don't stay tight with your head, the opponent will be able to push your head away, making it difficult to finish.

There are many ways to finish the single-leg takedown once you have your opponent's leg. This section covers four of the most common and effective finishes.

Run the pipe

While holding on firmly to your opponent's leg, take three or four quick steps backward. If he doesn't hop toward you, he will be in a stretched out, near-split position. While he is off balance, circle counterclockwise by stepping back with your left leg and driving your right shoulder into his right thigh. He will have no way to post a hand or leg behind him, and will be forced onto his back. Make sure to step back quickly and turn hard so that your opponent doesn't have time to adjust and catch his balance.

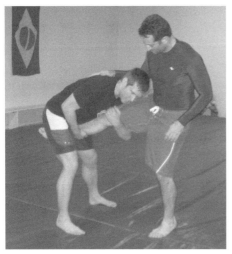

Figure 89.
Run the pipe, start.

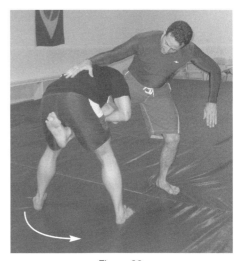

Figure 90.
Run the pipe, circle.

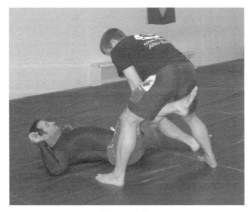

Figure 91.
Run the pipe, finish.

Flare

Your opponent will sometimes be able to get his lower leg free and bring it to your left side as shown in Figure 93. If this happens, take a deep step across the front of his body with your left leg, lift up on his left leg with your left hand, and block his knee with your right hand. The knee block doesn't have to be forceful, but it is intended to prevent him from hopping to the side. The opponent should land on his side, as demonstrated. A common error in the flare is attempting to drive the opponent toward his back rather than toward his side.

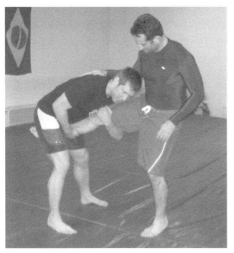

Figure 92.
Flare, start.

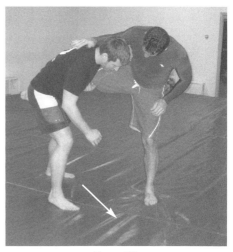

Figure 93.
Flare, lower leg free.

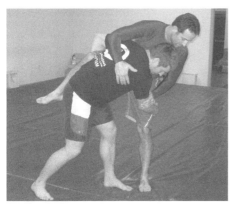

Figure 94.
Flare, step and knee block.

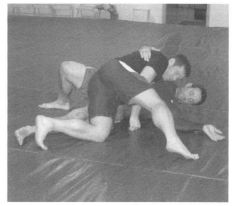

Figure 95.
Flare, finish.

Grappling Basics: A New Twist on Conditioning | 31

Backward trip

If the opponent brings the leg you are holding to the front of your body, switch your grip so that your left hand is near his ankle. Lift up on his ankle and leg as high as you can with both arms and walk forward to get your opponent on his toes. Suddenly switch directions and pull the opponent in a circle while blocking his grounded ankle with your right foot. He will fall onto his back.

A common problem when executing the backward trip is not lifting up on the leg as you turn the opponent. Lifting will keep your opponent off balance so he will be less able to defend the takedown.

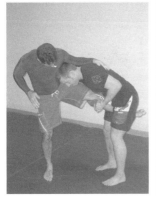 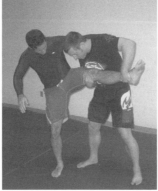 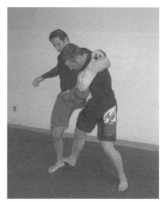

Figures 96–98.
Backward trip, ankle block.

Ankle pick

Begin the ankle pick with a head and wrist tie-up as shown in Figure 99 (to review, see page 22). Pull your opponent forward with both arms and take a circular step with your left leg. This move will usually cause him to step forward with his right leg to catch his balance. As soon as he puts all his weight onto his right foot, drive his head down and toward that foot. Release the grip on the wrist, grab the opponent's ankle, and execute a penetration step. Drive all the way through, and your opponent will end up on his right side.

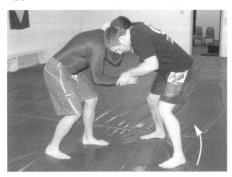 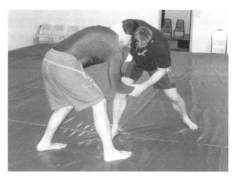

Figure 99.
Ankle pick, start.

Figure 100.
Ankle pick, drive down.

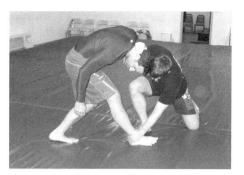
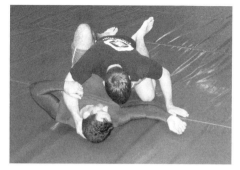

Figure 101.
Ankle pick, ankle grab.

Figure 102.
Ankle pick, penetration step and finish.

The most common mistake in this throw is not loading all of the opponent's weight on the foot that you are attacking. If he can lift it off the mat, the throw will not work. Be sure that when you drop toward his foot, you pull the opponent's head down with you.

Hip toss

Set up the hip toss from a head and elbow tie-up (see page 24). Get your hips into position by stepping across with your right leg and pivoting on both feet as shown in Figures 103 and 104. Hug the opponent's head tightly with your right arm and pull the elbow tight to your chest with the left arm. Drop your hips down several inches by bending at the knees to pull the opponent onto you. Then drive off the balls of your feet and twist your upper body. When first learning the move, throw the opponent and let him land in front of you. As you become more proficient and develop better control, throw him and land in the scarf hold (see page 49).

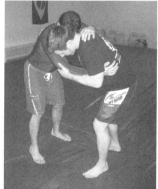
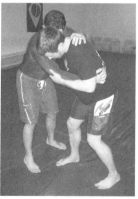

Figures 103 and 104.
Hip toss, step across and pivot.

Figure 105.
Hip toss, head hug, elbow pull, and hip drop.

Grappling Basics: A New Twist on Conditioning | 33

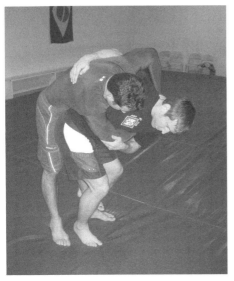

Figure 106.
Hip toss, upper body twist.

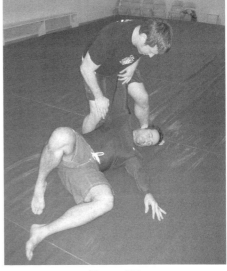

Figure 107.
Hip toss, finish.

One of the most common errors is stepping too far into your opponent and knocking him backward with your hips. Make sure to step *in front of* him rather than *into* him. The opponent should be on his toes rather than on his heels when you are in position to finish the throw. Another problem is not bending enough at the knees to get under the opponent. Although a slight bend at the waist is necessary, most of the drop in your hips is from the knee bend. Attempting to throw with straight legs, as shown in Figure 108, is nearly impossible. Finally, be sure to twist your upper body to allow the opponent to go over your back. Look in the direction of the throw.

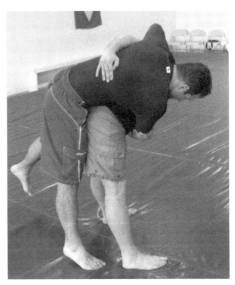

Figure 108.
Hip toss, incorrect position with straight legs.

Body-lock and trip

During a pummeling exchange, swim both arms inside as shown in Figure 109. Drop your level and step in as close as possible to your opponent. Bear hug him tightly around the waist and drive your shoulder into his chest to tip him off balance to the rear. Hook his left leg with your right leg and trip him backward. Stay close during the fall, only releasing the bear hug immediately before impact. You should land on top of your opponent.

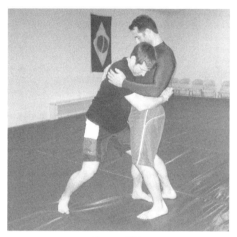

Figure 109.
Body-lock and trip, set-up.

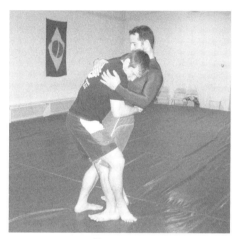

Figure 110.
Body-lock and trip, leg hook.

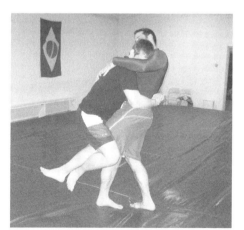

Figure 111.
Body-lock and trip, fall.

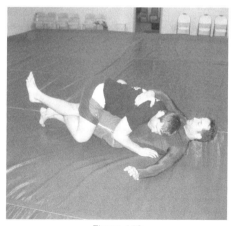

Figure 112.
Body-lock and trip, finish.

Grappling Basics: A New Twist on Conditioning | **35**

A common error involves attempting the trip with your body too far away from your opponent. Get chest to chest with your hips close before tripping, and never reach for the opponent's leg, as shown in Figure 114. This position makes it easy for the opponent to counter you.

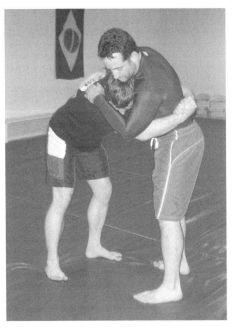 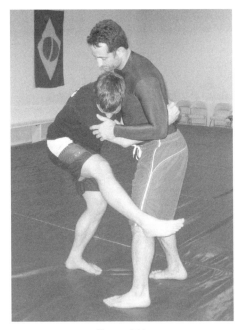

Figure 113.
Body-lock and trip, too far from opponent.

Figure 114.
Body-lock and trip, incorrect position reaching with leg.

Chapter 3

Ground Positioning and Pins

Once you get your opponent to the mat, you must be able to control him so that you can apply submission locks and defend against your opponent's attacks. Different grappling styles emphasize different aspects of matwork. For instance, in wrestling the goal is to pin your opponent's shoulders to the mat—and submission locks or chokes are not allowed. In judo, sambo, jiu-jitsu, and submission wrestling on the other hand, you may score from securing and maintaining dominant positions, but you can win instantly if you apply a joint lock or choke and cause your opponent to submit. This chapter covers the basic principles of positioning and pinning from the mat. The techniques covered are included because they are common to several different grappling styles and provide the beginner with a well-rounded foundation.

Overview of Positions

The basic ground positions covered in this chapter are: mount, cross side, scarf hold, back mount and guard. These positions are illustrated in Figures 115 through 119. For each position, a grappler may either be the top man or bottom man. It is important for all grapplers to become familiar with these positions, and the techniques and tactics appropriate to each one. Perhaps even more important than knowing the **how** (specific techniques) for each position is knowing the **what**—what is the goal. For example, a grappler who has the top position in the guard or who is stuck between the opponent's legs should know immediately that his goal is to break the legs open and escape to a better position (guard pass). If you don't have a basic plan of action, anything you do is undirected, wasted energy. Before you worry about the techniques, know what your course of action should be from each position. As you learn the techniques, you will be able to plug them into your overall game plan.

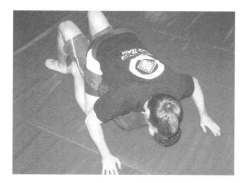

Figure 115.
Mount position (top).

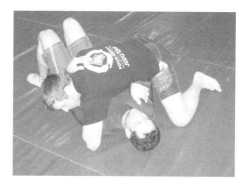

Figure 116.
Cross side position (top).

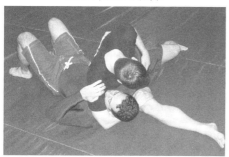

Figure 117.
Scarf hold position (top).

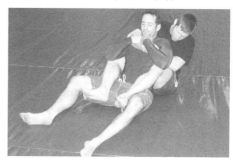

Figure 118.
Back mount position (bottom).

A central axiom in submission grappling is "position before submission." Submission techniques and making your opponent tap out may be more exciting than training positional skills, but if you aren't able to escape from disadvantageous positions and maintain dominant ones, you have almost no chance of applying a submission hold. Submission techniques require that you control your opponent long enough to apply them. Knowing a lot of arm locks and chokes is worthless if you cannot get into and hold the position required to use them. Therefore, it is imperative that you spend ample time training positional skills before concerning yourself with submissions.

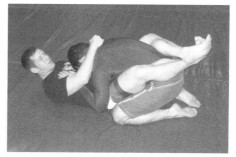

Figure 119.
Guard position (bottom).

Grappling Basics: A New Twist on Conditioning | **39**

Grappling positions are dynamic rather than static. Although they are classified according to several key features, your exact body placement will vary when the hold is applied. As your opponent attempts to escape, you must adjust your body accordingly to maintain control. Attempting to hold a rigid, static position while your opponent moves increases his chances of escaping. Several photos illustrate each position, but these are by no means an exhaustive catalog of possible variations in body placement.

Top game pressure

Controlling your opponent from the top requires that you keep your weight on him. As easy as this might sound, it takes substantial practice to be able to relax your body and let him carry all of your weight. Pressure is difficult to describe or illustrate. It is helpful to imagine that you are a bag of wet sand lying on top of your opponent. If he pushes with both hands as in a bench press, you must slide down between his hands by twisting your body. When working with a partner, have him give you feedback as to when you feel the heaviest to him. Notice how your body feels to you in that optimally heavy situation and remember it.

Training top game pressure without an opponent can be done with an inflatable ball or Swiss ball (a standard size ball of 55 or 65 cm will work). Place your chest on the ball and keep your hands in the air. Move around on the ball forward and backward and from side to side, even flipping over to your back, and keep your knees off the mat. Keep all of the force concentrated on the one spot that is touching the ball. Remember how this feels and try to recreate the sensation when you are grappling with an opponent.

Bottom game defense

With the exception of the guard, the bottom man is normally at a disadvantage and should look to defend and escape. When on the bottom, keep your arms bent and your elbows close to your sides to prevent any submissions. Straightening your arms, unless required for a specific technique, puts you at risk for arm locks. If possible, keep your hands near your neck to prevent chokes or to relieve pressure on your throat.

Try to keep moving when on the bottom. If you let your opponent settle into a tight top position, you will have to fight much harder to get out. Go from one escape attempt to the next so that your opponent will be off balance. It can be difficult to breathe when stuck on the bottom and many people get a sense of panic and claustrophobia. Although this is normal, you must work through it. Panic and its resultant wild flailing will not help you escape. Drill your bottom escapes frequently.

Another factor that differentiates superior versus inferior positional strategy is space. The grappler in the dominant position wants to eliminate space between himself and his opponent. This is done by dropping his weight to become heavier and locking up the head or limbs of the opponent. The bottom man must create space to escape by pushing and scooting away. Holding and gripping from the bottom is mostly wasted effort because it only keeps the opponent in the superior position.

Mount

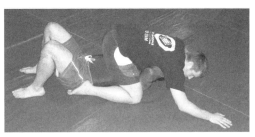

Figure 120.
High mount.

The mount position is one of the most dominant positions in grappling. In this position, your opponent is on his back and you are straddling his chest or hips. There are two basic mount positions: the high position, in which you are on the opponent's chest, and the low position, in which you are over the opponent's hips. In the high mount, you must keep your knees tight against your opponent's sides, your chest low, and at least one arm free to post on the mat when your opponent bridges or tries to buck you off (Figure 120).

High mount position
The basic techniques for holding the high mount are as follows:
- If the opponent bridges, use your arms to post on the mat.

- If he pushes up on your chest, as if bench pressing, swim your arms through, twist your body, and get your chest back down (Figures 121–124).

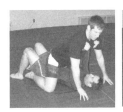 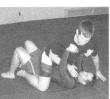 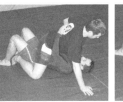 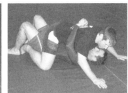

Figure 121.
Swim through, start.

Figures 122 and 123.
Swim through, swim arms and twist.

Figure 124.
Swim through, drop chest.

Grappling Basics: A New Twist on Conditioning | 41

- If he pushes on your knees, lift upward on his hands to slide them off (Figures 125–126). Alternatively, you can grab your opponent's wrists and lift up so that his hands slide off your knees.

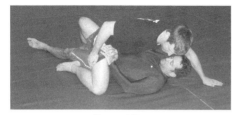

Figure 125.
High mount, hand push on knee.

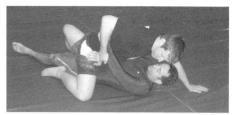

Figure 126.
High mount, pull up on wrist.

- If he pushes on your knees with his elbows, cup your hands under his elbows and lift up (Figures 127–128). This will cause his elbows to slip off and prevent him from pushing.

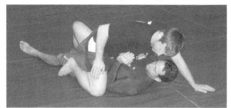

Figure 127.
High mount, elbow push on knee.

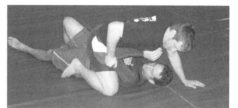

Figure 128.
High mount, pull up on elbow.

- If the opponent rolls to his side, don't stop him but rather take the position shown in Figure 129. From here you can return to the mount if he turns back; or if he continues to roll away, you can take his back.

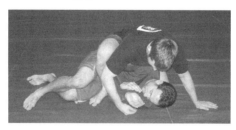

Figure 129.
High mount, opponent rolls to side.

Low mount position

For the low mount, keep your hips on top of your opponent, as shown. Your legs should be near his legs so that you can "grapevine"—or intertwine—your legs with his to maintain stability. Be sure to push your hips down and into the opponent. If he bridges, straighten your legs to flatten him out. In general, the low mount is an easier position to hold but gives you fewer submission opportunities than the high mount.

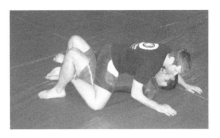

Figure 130.
Low mount.

Mount escapes

Trap and roll

When an opponent in the high mount puts his right arm behind your head and is high on your chest, he is in position for you to use this escape. Trap his right arm with your left arm as shown in Figure 132. Next, bring your left foot up to the outside of his right foot. Finally, bridge up and to the left, reaching with your right arm to push on his armpit. You should end up in your opponent's guard.

A common problem with this escape is trying to roll the opponent directly to the side without a strong bridge. Review the bridging drill on page 86 before learning this escape. Without first bridging, the opponent will be difficult to roll, particularly if he is heavier than you.

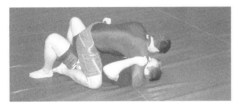

Figure 131.
Trap and roll escape, start.

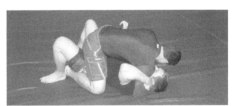

Figure 132.
Trap and roll escape, trap right arm, left foot to outside.

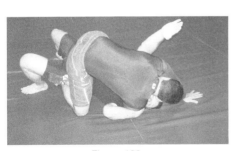

Figure 133.
Trap and roll escape, bridge and armpit push.

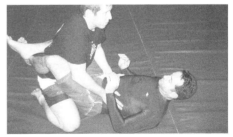

Figure 134.
Trap and roll escape, finish in opponent's guard.

Grappling Basics: A New Twist on Conditioning | **43**

Shrimp-out

The shrimp-out escape is based on the shrimp movement drill described in Chapter 5. First get onto your left side and put both hands on the opponent's right knee or thigh, as shown in Figure 135. Push with your arms as you bring your left knee toward your chest. Your left leg should slide under the opponent's right leg, as shown in Figure 136. Immediately lock your legs around the opponent's right leg. Next, turn to your right side and release your legs but maintain a hook on the opponent's right leg with your left leg (Figure 138). This prevents your opponent from freeing his leg as you finish the technique. Put both hands on the opponent's left knee or thigh and drag your right knee up to your chest. Lock your legs around him and establish the closed guard as in Figure 139.

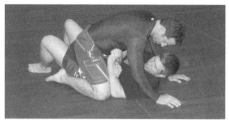

Figure 135.
Shrimp-out escape, start.

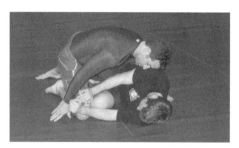

Figure 136.
Shrimp-out escape, left leg slide up.

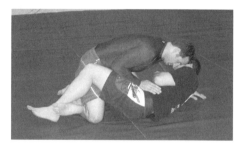

Figure 137.
Shrimp-out escape, leg lock.

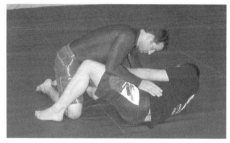

Figure 138.
Shrimp-out escape, turn and hook;
right leg drag.

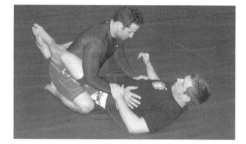

Figure 139.
Shrimp-out escape, finish in guard.

The most frequent problem with this escape is poor shrimping technique. Drill the shrimping movement (see page 76) without a partner until you are proficient. Get completely onto your side when executing the movement. If you are flat on your back, it will not work.

Hip bump

When the opponent is sitting on your hips, bring your elbows in and your hands to his hips. Next, bridge up and push him forward with your knee, causing him to fall forward and post both hands on the mat. Explosively bridge your hips up and lock your elbows out when the opponent is in the air. Drop your hips back to the mat, but keep your elbows locked to support the opponent. From here there are two options based on what your opponent does. If he has lost his balance and is falling, push him off and get up quickly (Figures 140–142). If he is still close to you, use the space created to draw your knees to your chest, scoot up and put him in your guard (Figures 143–146).

The most common problem with this technique is only attempting to press the opponent off you rather than using the power of your hips to elevate him as well. Remember that the arms are used as a support only.

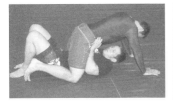
Figure 140.
Hip bump, elbows in, hands to hips.

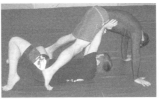
Figure 141.
Hip bump, bridge and push.

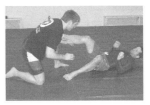
Figure 142.
Hip bump, finish and get up.

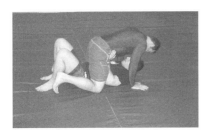
Figure 143.
Hip bump, start.

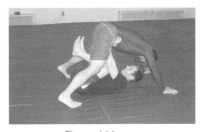
Figure 144.
Hip bump, knees to chest.

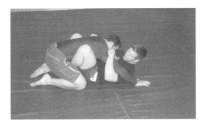
Figure 145.
Hip bump, scoot up.

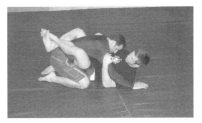
Figure 146.
Hip bump, finish in guard.

Grappling Basics: A New Twist on Conditioning | **45**

Cross Side

The cross side position is a common control position in which the top grappler is lying chest to chest, with his body perpendicular or nearly perpendicular (crosswise) to the bottom grappler's. We will cover three basic cross side variations.

In the first variation, shown in Figure 147, the top grappler has both of his arms on one side of the opponent's body and both knees on the other. To hold this position from the top, you must maintain chest contact and keep your weight on your opponent. Pinch your knees and elbows in tightly to his sides.

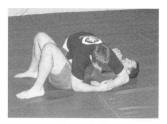

Figure 147.
Cross side variation,
both arms on one side.

The second position involves keeping one hand by the near-side hip and the other hand by the far-side hip (Figure 148). The top grappler's legs are stretched out and the hips dropped down to increase the pressure. To hold this position, you must use your left arm to prevent the bottom grappler from rolling away, and your right hand to prevent him from raising his right knee and putting you in the guard.

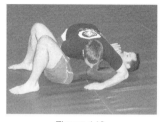

Figure 148.
Cross side variation,
hands on each side.

In the third position, one arm is under your opponent's head and neck while the other is blocking the hip on the side closest to you.

As the opponent pushes on your hip with his right arm, you may need to switch your hips. During this movement, keep your chest in contact with your opponent's. Lift up on the opponent's right shoulder and arm, and switch your hips back and forth between the two positions shown in Figures 150 and 151.

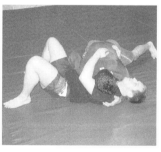

Figure 149.
Cross side variation, arm under
neck and hip block.

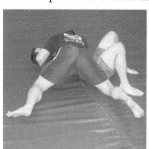 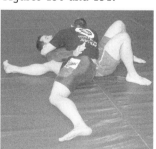

Figures 150 and 151.
Cross side hip switch.

Cross side escapes

<u>Shrimp-out</u>

When the opponent has both arms across your body as in Figure 152, the shrimp-out movement works well. Bridge up into the opponent and drop down quickly; post on the opponent's hip with your right hand, and bring your right knee inside as shown in Figures 153 and 154. Your knee should be between your and your opponent's chests. From here, push your body away so that you can pull your whole leg toward your chest and put the opponent in the guard, as shown in Figures 155 and 156.

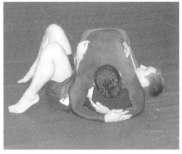

A common mistake is not bridging high enough and dropping fast enough to get your knee in. Without a high bridge and fast drop you won't have enough space. Also, be sure to immediately extend your body so that you can get into the guard position; otherwise, the opponent will just circle around and regain cross side.

Figure 152.
Shrimp-out escape
from cross side, start.

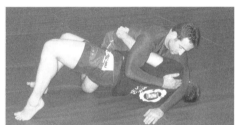
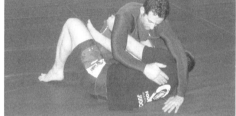

Figures 153 and 154.
Shrimp-out escape from cross side, bridge and knee lift.

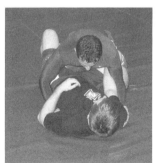
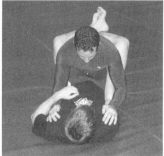

Figures 155 and 156.
Shrimp-out escape from cross side, finish in guard.

Grappling Basics: A New Twist on Conditioning | 47

Bridge and roll

If the opponent has one hand behind your head and the other by your hip, you can bridge and roll him. First, set him up with a hard bridge toward him. You have to really exaggerate this motion. When he pushes back, bear hug his body; then drop down and bridge hard in the other direction. Timing and energy are everything in this technique. If the opponent is not pushing into you, it is almost impossible to bridge him over. However, if the opponent is not resisting your bridge, you can usually go immediately into the shrimp-out.

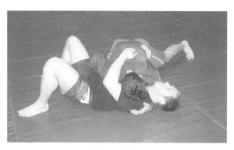

Figure 157.
Bridge and roll, start.

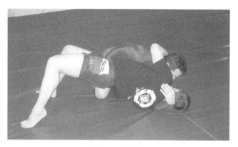

Figure 158.
Bridge and roll, hard bridge toward opponent.

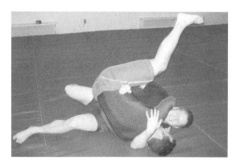

Figure 159.
Bridge and roll, bear hug and bridge to other side.

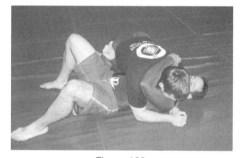

Figure 160.
Bridge and roll, finish in cross side

The main problem most grapplers encounter with this technique is that they do not bridge properly. Make sure that you are bridging the opponent up and over rather than just rolling. Practice with a partner heavier than you, and you will know if your technique is sound.

Belly down

This cross side escape begins with a bridge. At the top of the bridge, push with both arms on the opponent and thread your right leg under your left leg to spin out to your stomach, as shown in Figure 163. You must keep the left foot planted. Move your right leg away from your opponent (Figure 164). Keep your arms locked to prevent the opponent from coming toward you.

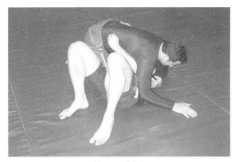
Figure 161.
Belly down escape, start.

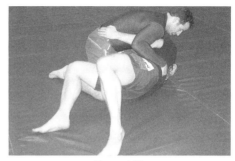
Figure 162.
Belly down escape, bridge and push.

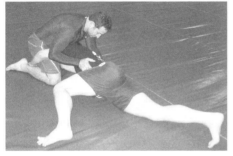
Figure 163.
Belly down escape, thread leg and spin out.

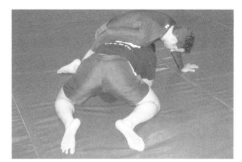
Figure 164.
Belly down escape, finish on stomach.

The main problem that most grapplers encounter when learning this technique is that they try to turn into the opponent instead of pushing away from him. If you are having trouble you can practice the technique against a wall.

Scarf Hold

The scarf hold (so named because of the translation from the Japanese *kesa gatame*) is a basic control position used in many different types of grappling. To perform the scarf hold, grab the opponent's head with your right arm and hug tightly. Pull the opponent's right arm across your body with your left arm, holding it tightly at the elbow. Split your legs apart for maximum balance and sink your weight down onto your opponent's chest as shown in Figure 165.

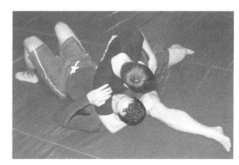
Figure 165.
Scarf hold.

Grappling Basics: A New Twist on Conditioning | **49**

As the opponent moves, it is important to move with him so that you maintain the same position relative to him. If he spins in a circle, move just enough so that you maintain a constant position. Keep your legs away from his so that he can't trap them and escape. As the opponent bucks and twists to throw you off, keep your weight down as much as possible.

Scarf hold escapes

<u>Bridge and roll</u>
The most basic escape from the scarf hold is the bridge and roll. To perform this move, you need to create some resistance from your opponent. First, bridge into him as hard as you can as shown in Figure 167. If his hold is not solid, this alone may get you out; however, usually it will cause the opponent to drive into you in an attempt to flatten you out. When you feel the opponent drive, drop your body back to the floor, bear hug him, and bridge in the opposite direction. His own momentum combined with your bridge should send him over easily, as shown in Figure 168.

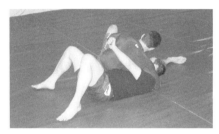

Figure 166.
Bridge and roll, start.

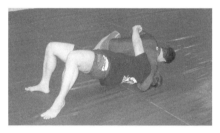

Figure 167.
Bridge and roll, hard bridge into opponent.

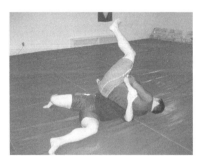

Figure 168.
Bridge and roll, bear hug and bridge to other side.

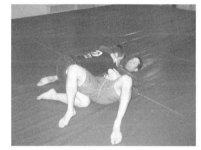

Figure 169.
Bridge and roll, finish in cross side position.

Most problems with this technique come with a poorly-executed or ill-timed bridge. You must bridge as hard as possible into the opponent to provoke a reaction; otherwise, the opponent will be much too heavy to roll. You must also switch immediately into the second bridge before your opponent can recover his balance.

Twist out

For this escape you must create some momentum using your legs. Cross your ankles and swing your legs from side to side to get your opponent moving, as shown in Figure 170. He will be forced to move in order to maintain the pin. After a few swings, twist hard into the opponent and pull your right arm out as your legs move toward him (Figure 171). This motion must be as explosive as possible. If your arm only comes out part way, repeat the twist until you are behind your opponent (Figure 172). To release the grip on the head, place your left palm flat on the mat and look up. This will put pressure on your opponent's shoulder and cause him to release.

Motion and momentum are the keys to this escape. If you have problems with it, you most likely need to move more. Keep your ankles crossed so that all of your lower-body weight moves at once. Be persistent if the move doesn't immediately work. No one said it would be *easy* to get out of the pin, just *possible*.

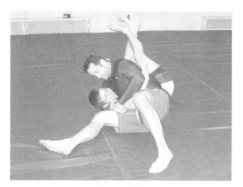

Figure 170.
Scarf hold twist out, leg swing.

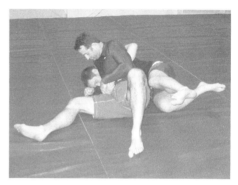

Figure 171.
Scarf hold twist out, twist into opponent.

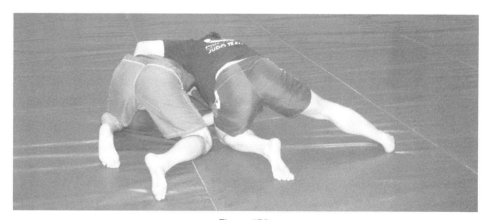

Figure 172.
Scarf hold twist out, finish.

Grappling Basics: A New Twist on Conditioning | 51

Back Mount

The value of the back mount position depends on which style of grappling you practice. In wrestling and judo, spinning to your stomach, or "turtling," can make it difficult for your opponent to pin or attack you. Therefore the back mount position is of limited use because it makes a pin easier. However, in submission wrestling or jiu-jitsu, points are given for obtaining a back mount, and you have a wide range of submission attacks available.

The back mount is accomplished by wrapping your legs around your opponent and hooking your feet on his inner thighs (known as "putting in your hooks"), as shown in Figure 173. Your arms are around his neck or chest and are used to control him or apply submission holds. Whether your opponent is face down or face up, the key is to keep your chest facing his back. If he turns, you must turn with him. Staying still as he twists will let him escape into the guard.

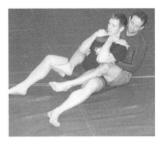

Figure 173.
Back mount position.

Back mount escapes

When your opponent gets a back mount on you, you must first bring up your hands to protect your neck from chokes, as shown in Figure 173. If the back mount is poorly applied and the opponent doesn't put his hooks in, just dip your head, raise your hips, and roll him off.

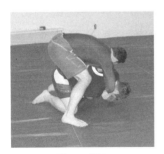

Figure 174.
Back mount escape without hooks, dip head and roll.

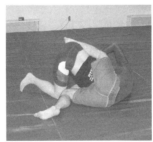

Figure 175.
Back mount escape without hooks, raise hips.

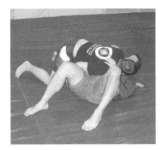

Figure 176.
Back mount escape without hooks, finish in cross side.

If the hooks are in, escaping from the position shown in Figure 177 is difficult. Try to roll so that your opponent's back is on the mat. If the opponent is attempting a choke, block it by pulling down on his arm with both hands. Roll to the side away from the elbow of his choking hand, as shown in Figure 178. Going toward the elbow will only tighten up his hold. When you are on your side, remove the left hook by kicking your left leg straight, and then quickly putting it on top of your opponent's leg (Figure 179). Keep his leg trapped as you scoot your whole body to the left (Figure 180). Make sure you are scooting with your chest facing up, rather than rolling. If you roll, your opponent can put the hook back in. Once you have scooted out until your butt is on the mat (Figure 181), twist back into your opponent, as shown in Figure 182. Depending on the situation, you may end up in the guard or cross side position. In the worst case, your opponent may move more quickly and mount you, but this situation is still better than a back mount.

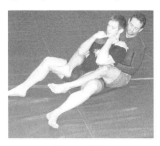
Figure 177.
Back mount escape, block choke.

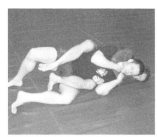
Figure 178.
Back mount escape, roll away.

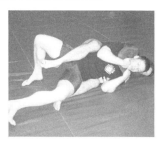
Figure 179.
Back mount escape, remove hook.

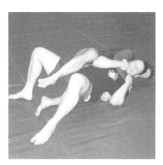
Figure 180.
Back mount escape, body scoot.

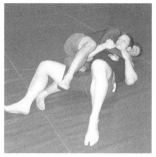
Figure 181.
Back mount escape, butt on mat.

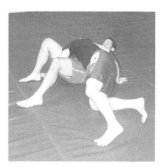
Figure 182.
Back mount escape, twist.

Most people have trouble with the back mount escape at first because there are so many important steps. Train slowly and methodically until it becomes fluid. Only then should you speed up and have the opponent offer resistance. This technique will not work if the opponent has his ankles crossed, but you may be able to submit him or get him to uncross them by using the ankle lock technique shown in Chapter 4.

Grappling Basics: A New Twist on Conditioning | **53**

Guard

The guard is a position in which one grappler is on his back and the other is trapped between or entangled in the bottom man's legs. If the bottom grappler has his ankles crossed, as in Figure 183, it is called a closed guard. If his legs are open as in Figure 184, it is known as an open guard. When discussing the techniques, we will say that the bottom man has the guard and the top man is in the guard.

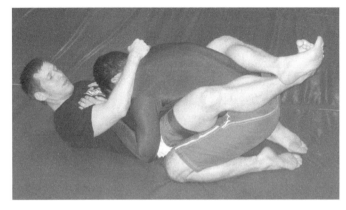

Figure 183.
Closed guard.

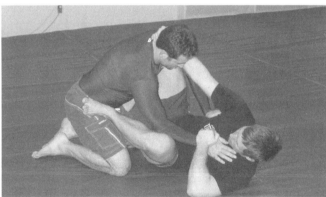

Figure 184.
Open guard.

The guard is different from most other grappling ground situations in that the bottom man is actually in control when he has the guard. He is not being pinned even though he is on the bottom because his legs allow him to control the top man's body and to apply various offensive techniques. The bottom grappler may either sweep or submit his opponent. A sweep is a technique that puts the top man on his back and allows the bottom man to get the top position. Submissions, covered in the next chapter, force the other grappler to tap out or give up. The top grappler, who is in the guard, must try to pass the guard and get into a pinning position, such as cross side or mount.

Guard – bottom position

The grappler in the bottom position of the guard has the advantage. If you are on the bottom, maintain control of your opponent by locking your ankles and getting a grip on your opponent's head and/or arms. Some different grip positions are shown in Figures 185 and 186. Having your opponent in the guard is only an advantage if you use it to your benefit by attempting sweeps or submission holds. Simply gripping him and hanging on is a stalling tactic that can be quickly overcome by an experienced opponent.

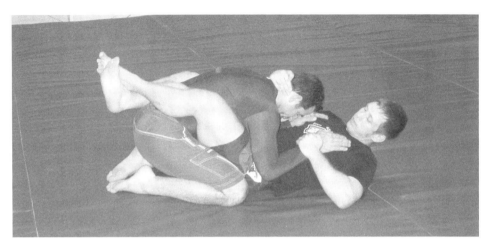

Figure 185.
Guard position, head lock.

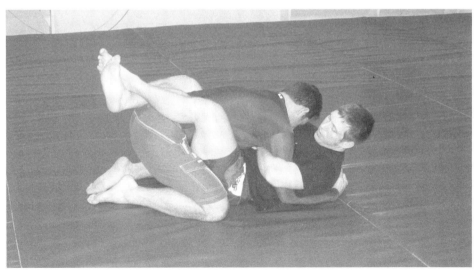

Figure 186.
Guard position, arm lock.

Guard sweeps

<u>Scissors sweep</u>

To apply the scissors sweep, grip the opponent's head and arm as shown in Figure 187. Open your legs and turn onto your left side. Your left leg should be on the mat and your right shin should be on the opponent's stomach, as shown in Figure 188. Pull the opponent forward using your arms and make a scissor motion with your legs. Your left leg slides across the floor to push on the opponent's right leg, and your right leg pushes on the opponent's hip (Figure 189). Follow the opponent over and take the mount position.

One problem in applying this technique is not pulling the opponent into you. Get more power by stretching your body out as you pull. If your opponent stays seated and balanced, you will not be able to sweep him. It will also be difficult to make this technique work if you do not scissor your legs powerfully.

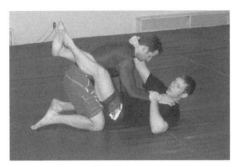

Figure 187.
Scissors sweep, start.

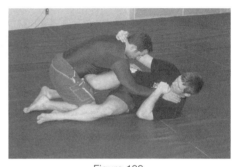

Figure 188.
Scissors sweep, turn and shin to stomach.

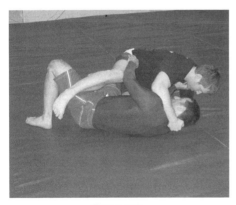

Figure 189.
Scissors sweep, scissor legs, push on hip.

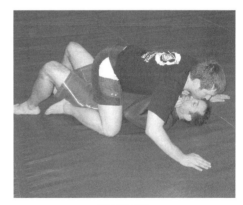

Figure 190.
Scissors sweep, finish in mount.

Sit-up sweep

When you have the guard and are attempting to control your opponent and pull him close to you, he will often defend by posturing up and pulling away. The sit-up sweep uses his momentum against him. As the opponent pulls away, drop your left hand and post it on the floor, as shown in Figure 191. Open your legs and drop both feet to the mat. Reach across his body with your right hand and place it on his right elbow as shown in Figure 193. Push off with your right foot and your left arm, drive your hips forward, and rotate him to the left and onto his back as shown in Figure 194. You should end up in the mount position.

It is important to apply this technique when the opponent is pulling away. If you try this sweep when he is driving into you, it will not work. Be sure to control his right elbow with your right hand so that he cannot post it and block the sweep.

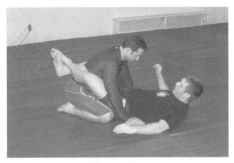

Figure 191.
Sit-up sweep, start.

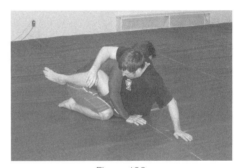

Figure 192.
Sit-up sweep, post arm and open legs.

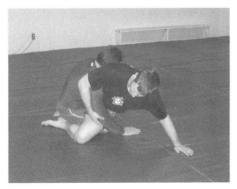

Figure 193.
Sit-up sweep, elbow control and push off.

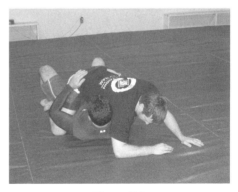

Figure 194.
Sit-up sweep, rotate into mount.

Grappling Basics: A New Twist on Conditioning | 57

Guard passing

When you are on top, trapped in your opponent's guard, your main goal is to pass the guard. Passing involves forcing your opponent to unlock his legs, and then moving around his legs into a control position, such as a mount or cross side. Attempting submission attacks from within an opponent's guard is not recommended. Not only will these attacks usually fail, but they will also put you off balance and allow your opponent to sweep or submit you.

The first step in any guard-passing attempt is to get into a balanced position often referred to as "posture." Just as in Figure 195, you should be sitting with your butt on your heels, head up, and elbows tucked in. Make sure you are not leaning forward, backward, or to either side. Practice maintaining this position with your partner pushing and pulling you with his arms and legs as a preliminary guard-passing drill.

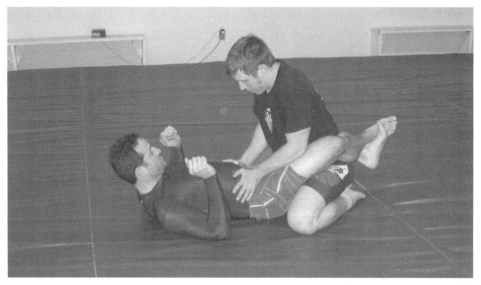

Figure 195.
Posture for guard passing.

Breaking the guard

If the opponent has closed his guard, you will first have to break it open before you can pass the guard. Bring your elbows to the inside of the opponent's thighs and place your hands on his hip bones, as shown in Figure 196. Widen your base by sliding your right knee away, and drop your body while pressing your elbows into his inner thighs. When done properly, this technique will cause enough discomfort to force the opponent to open his legs. Once his legs open, immediately bring one knee up, as shown in Figure 198, to prevent him from reestablishing a closed guard.

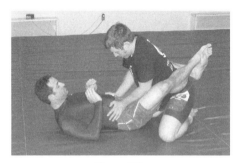

Figure 196.
Breaking the guard, elbows to inner thighs.

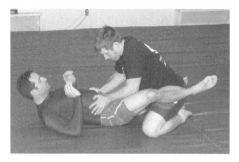

Figure 197.
Breaking the guard, widen base and press elbows.

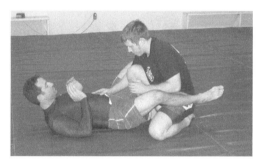

Figure 198.
Breaking the guard, knee up.

Remember that the purpose of this technique is to open the legs, not to force a submission. Once the legs come open, you must stop the elbow press and get into position. Practice will build an immediate awareness of when the legs come open.

Grappling Basics: A New Twist on Conditioning | 59

Leg throw

For the leg throw, you will be standing while your partner is on his back, as shown in Figure 199. This situation could happen after a takedown or a guard break. Grab his ankles with your hands to control his legs, and make a faking motion as if you were going to throw his legs to your right side; instead, suddenly switch and throw them to the left. Step your right foot beside your partner's left hip, and bring your left foot up into a stable stance, as shown in Figure 201. From here you can kneel down and pin him in a cross side hold (Figure 202). The goal is not to throw your opponent's legs far, but to just clear them so that you can step around—the emphasis is on speed rather than power.

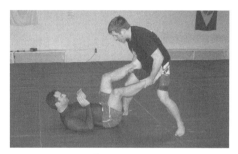

Figure 199.
Leg throw, start.

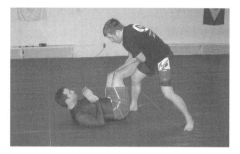

Figure 200.
Leg throw, fake throw.

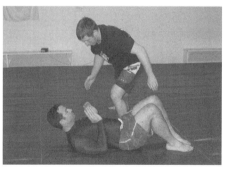

Figure 201.
Leg throw, stable foot position.

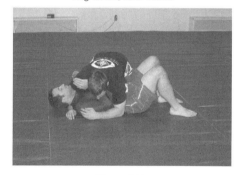

Figure 202.
Leg throw, finish in cross side.

Single underhook

To practice the single underhook, get into a kneeling position and swim your left arm under your opponent's right leg and pin his left leg in the crook of his knee with your right hand. Make sure that your opponent's right leg is up on your left shoulder, as shown in Figure 204. Reach across your opponent's body with your left arm, grab his left shoulder, and drive your weight into him, as shown in Figure 205. Walk your body to your left and drop your left shoulder toward the mat so that his leg slides off and you end up in the cross side position, as shown in Figure 207.

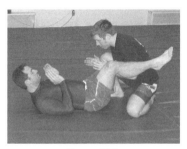

Figure 203.
Single underhook, start.

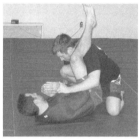

Figure 204.
Single underhook, swim and leg pin.

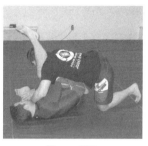

Figure 205.
Single underhook, reach and weight drive.

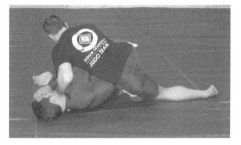

Figure 206.
Single underhook, walk and shoulder drop.

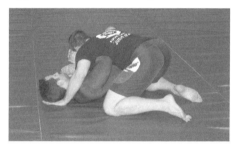

Figure 207.
Single underhook, finish in cross side.

It is important that you keep your weight down on your opponent so that he remains pinned during this technique. Also, make sure your right hand keeps your opponent's left leg pinned until you get around; otherwise you may be pulled into a triangle choke, as shown in Figure 208.

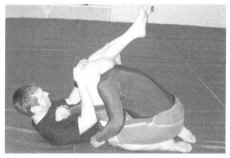

Figure 208.
Triangle choke.

Grappling Basics: A New Twist on Conditioning | 61

Double underhook

To practice the double underhook, start from the kneeling position and swim both arms under your opponent's legs, as shown in Figure 209. Cup your hands on his thighs and slide him toward you and onto his shoulders (Figure 211). Lock your hands together and keep downward pressure to pin him. Next, move to your left and twist your body so that your left shoulder drops down toward the mat. Allow the opponent's legs to fall down so that you end up in the cross side position, as shown in Figure 213. As with the single underhook pass, you must keep your weight down on your opponent throughout the drill.

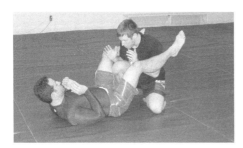

Figure 209.
Double underhook, swim.

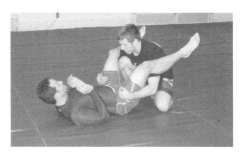

Figure 210.
Double underhook, cup and slide.

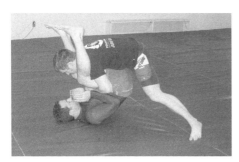

Figure 211.
Double underhook, downward pressure.

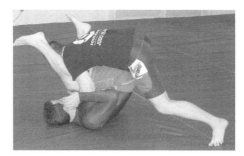

Figure 212.
Double underhook, twist and drop.

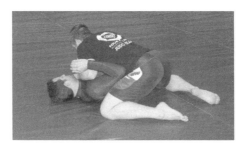

Figure 213.
Double underhook, finish in cross side.

Grappling Basics: A New Twist on Conditioning

Chapter

Submission

Submission techniques are designed to get the opponent to "tap out" or "submit," or in other words, to admit defeat by tapping the mat. Submission techniques generally fall into one of three categories: joint locks, chokes, or pain compliance. Joint locks (arm bars and leg locks) use leverage to place joints at risk of damage, and when an opponent realizes he cannot escape, he taps out. In competition, locks are applied with control so that the opponent has an opportunity to give up and avoid injury. In self-defense, the same lock applied with power and speed is used to damage the joint and disable an assailant.

Choking techniques compress the arteries and/or windpipe, cutting off oxygen to the brain. In competition, an opponent will tap out when he realizes there is no escape. In self-defense, the same technique can be held slightly longer to cause unconsciousness.

Finally, pain compliance techniques use leverage, pressure points, or other methods to cause extreme pain to an opponent. If applied in such a way that the opponent cannot escape, he will submit. Of the three types of submissions, pain compliance moves are the least reliable. Pain tolerance varies from person to person and may be influenced by adrenaline, alcohol, or other drugs. Although submission holds that cause pain will work, it is best not to rely on them.

Submission holds are not allowed in some grappling styles, such as wrestling. In other styles, the types of locks allowed or the parts of the body that can be attacked may be different. For example in judo, grapplers may use chokes or arm locks, but not leg locks. Sambo, on the other hand, incorporates certain leg locks but prohibits chokes in sport competition.

Joint Locks

Armbars

<u>Cross armbar</u>
This technique locks the elbow joint, forcing the elbow into hyperextension. Start the technique from the mounted position. When the opponent attempts to escape by pushing on your chest, place both hands on your opponent's chest and make a frame around his right arm, as shown in Figure 215. Transfer your weight to your hands so that you can spin to the side and put your left leg over the opponent's head. Your butt should be as close as possible to the opponent's right shoulder. Hold his right arm by hooking your left arm on his wrist or forearm and hold near the elbow with the right hand (Figure 217). Keep your knees pinched tightly together and lie back. Finish the lock by raising your hips slightly.

The cross armbar is a complex but fundamental move in submission grappling. The first problem most grapplers encounter when learning the move is lying back before placing the leg over the opponent's head. Doing this allows him to roll up into you and escape. Another problem is sitting too far from the opponent. If the opponent's elbow slips past your thighs, as in Figure 219, you will not be able to apply the lock. Finally, it is important to keep your knees pinched tightly together so that the opponent cannot twist his arm to the left or right and escape.

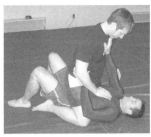
Figure 214.
Cross armbar, start.

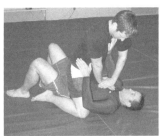
Figure 215.
Cross armbar, frame.

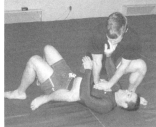
Figure 216.
Cross armbar, spin.

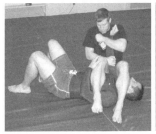
Figure 217.
Cross armbar, leg over head and arm hold.

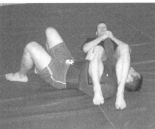
Figure 218.
Cross armbar, squeeze legs and lie back.

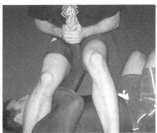
Figure 219.
Cross armbar, incorrect, sitting too far back

Guard armbar

The straight arm lock can also be applied from the guard. Clamp down on the opponent's right arm with your right arm. Your forearm should pinch his arm tightly to your chest and your hand should be behind his elbow. Place your left forearm on his neck with your left hand cupped behind his head, as shown in Figure 220. Push his head away and pivot your hips (Figure 221). Swing your left leg over his head as shown in Figure 222, pinch your knees together, pull your heels toward your butt, and extend your hips. Control his right arm at the wrist and at the elbow so he can't pull or twist out.

A key point of this technique that commonly causes problems is not controlling the opponent's arm tightly enough. Without arm control, your opponent will simply pull away as you pivot for the lock. Another problem area is in the hip pivot itself. Notice in Figure 220 how the bottom man begins the technique straight on with his opponent. At the conclusion of the technique as shown in Figure 223, he is completely perpendicular to the opponent. As you spin to your right, kick your right leg up into the opponent's armpit.

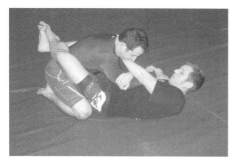

Figure 220.
Guard armbar, arm clamp.

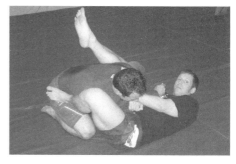

Figure 221.
Guard armbar, head push and pivot.

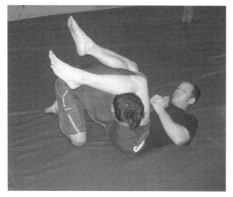

Figure 222.
Guard armbar, leg swing and arm control.

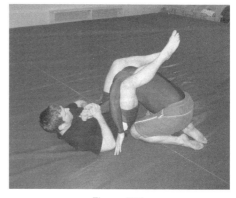

Figure 223.
Guard armbar, finish, view from other side; leg in armpit.

Bent arm lock (guard)

The bent arm lock, sometimes called the *kimura*, applies torque to the shoulder. It can be applied from the guard position when the opponent places his hand on the mat. Grab the opponent's left wrist with your right hand, as shown in Figure 224. Sit up and reach over his left arm with your left arm to grab your own right wrist, as shown in Figure 225. Scoot your hips out toward the opponent's arm and pull the opponent's left elbow close to your chest. Make sure to keep your ankles crossed, as shown in Figure 226, so that the opponent cannot escape by rolling forward. Finish the lock by twisting the opponent's arm toward the left.

A common error in this lock is not scooting your hips out far enough when you apply pressure to the shoulder. Staying directly in front of the opponent rather than to the side makes it much more difficult to finish. Also, be sure to keep your ankles together so that the opponent cannot roll out of the lock.

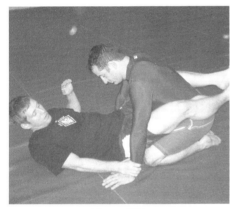

Figure 224.
Bent arm lock from guard, wrist grab.

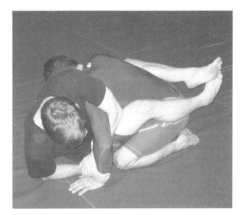

Figure 225.
Bent arm lock from guard, reach over, grab own wrist.

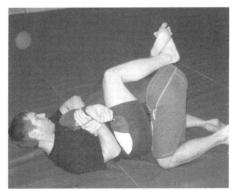

Figure 226.
Bent arm lock from guard, hip scoot and arm twist.

Grappling Basics: A New Twist on Conditioning | **67**

Bent arm lock (cross side)

You can also apply the bent arm lock described above when you are holding your opponent in the cross side position. Hug the opponent's left arm tightly to his side with your legs. Grab the opponent's right wrist with your right hand and push it down toward the mat as you reach under the opponent's arm; grip your own right wrist with your left hand, as shown in Figure 227. Finish the lock by dragging the opponent's elbow toward his side, and then rotating his elbow up and toward his head in a semi-circular motion.

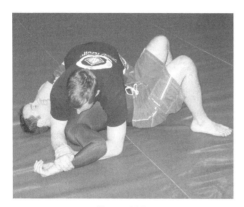

Figure 227.
Bent arm lock from cross side, wrist grab and pin.

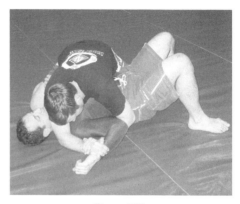

Figure 228.
Bent arm lock from cross side, drag and rotate elbow.

A common error with this technique is forgetting to drag the opponent's elbow toward his side before rotating the shoulder. If you forget, you will have to rotate the shoulder before he feels pressure in the shoulder, giving him a better chance to escape. Another common problem is taking your weight off the opponent when attempting the finish. Keep your chest in contact with his so that the pin is maintained throughout the technique.

Leg locks

Achilles lock

The Achilles lock is so named because pressure is applied to the ankle on the Achilles tendon. This lock causes pain from tendon compression and hyperextends the opponent's foot. When you are standing and your opponent is on his back attempting to fight from his guard, get control of his right foot with your left arm, as shown in Figure 229. Bend your right leg, and place your shin near his groin; put your left foot on his right hip and lie back on your right side (Figure 231). Pinch your knees together tightly. Grip his ankle, as in Figure 232, with the bone of your left forearm just above his right heel and his foot tucked into your armpit.

Grab your right wrist with your left hand and place the other hand on his shin. Apply pressure to his ankle by arching your back, pulling up with your left forearm, and pressing down with your right hand.

The Achilles lock is sometimes a difficult technique for beginners because they take an incorrect grip on the ankle. Study the photos and ask your training partner if the grip is tight. Keeping control of the opponent's leg is important, so your knees must remain tightly pinched. Finally, keep your left foot at the opponent's hip so that you can prevent him from sitting up into you and escaping.

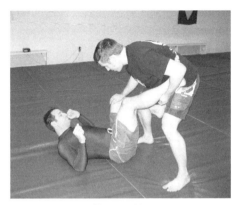

Figure 229.
Achilles lock, foot control.

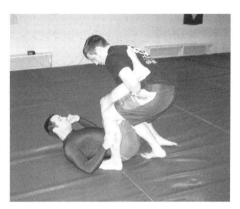

Figure 230.
Achilles lock, leg bend.

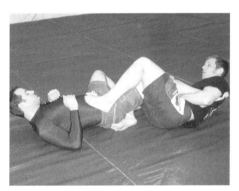

Figure 231.
Achilles lock, foot on hip, lie back.

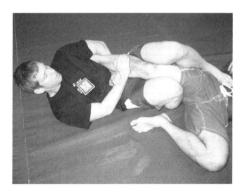

Figure 232.
Achilles lock, ankle grip and pressure.

Chokes

<u>Rear naked choke</u>

The rear naked choke (RNC) got its name from judo because it was one of the few chokes applied without the use of the *gi*, or uniform. To apply the choke, you must first get behind your opponent in the back mount position. Wrap your right arm around his neck so that the crook of your elbow is in front of his windpipe. Grab the biceps of your left arm with your right hand and put your left hand behind the opponent's head, as shown in Figure 234. Apply pressure using a hugging motion. Most of the pressure for the choke comes from your traps and back rather than your arms. Pulling with the arms is not only less powerful but can quickly lead to fatigue if you don't have the correct arm position.

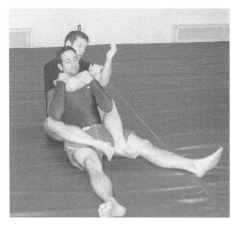
Figure 233.
Rear naked choke, biceps grab.

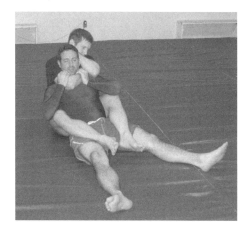
Figure 234.
Rear naked choke, hand behind head.

<u>Triangle choke</u>

In the triangle choke, you use your legs to choke your opponent. When your opponent is in your guard, grab both of his wrists. Simultaneously pull his right wrist and push his left wrist, as shown in Figure 235, as you open your legs. Clamp your legs down again with your right leg over his shoulder. Push your opponent's right arm toward your right side. Grab your right shin with your left hand and put your left foot on the opponent's hip (Figure 238). Push with your left leg to scoot your body to your right. Bring your left leg up and put your right instep in the crook of your left knee. Squeeze your knees together and clamp your heels toward your butt in a "cannonball" motion while pulling down on the opponent's head to make him submit, as shown in Figure 239.

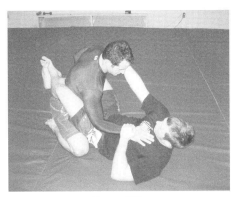

Figure 235.
Triangle choke, wrist grab, push and pull.

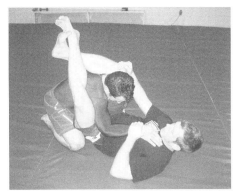

Figure 236.
Triangle choke, leg over shoulder.

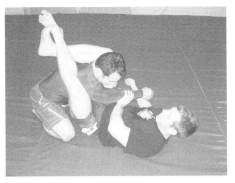

Figure 237.
Triangle choke, pull wrist across.

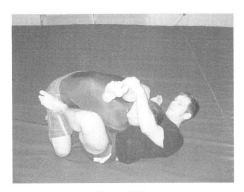

Figure 238.
Triangle choke, hand on shin, foot on hip.

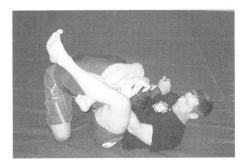

Figure 239.
Triangle choke, instep behind knee and squeeze.

The key to the triangle is to stay tight. The choke works by pushing the opponent's right shoulder into his neck on one side and your hamstring into his neck on the other side. Most errors result from leaving too much space between your legs and the opponent's neck. As you clamp down and make the turn, be sure that the legs stay tight.

Grappling Basics: A New Twist on Conditioning | **71**

Arm triangle

The arm triangle is a quick choke from the guard based on the same principles as the triangle done with the legs. When your opponent is in your guard and posts his right arm on your chest or neck, push it across your body with your left hand and pull him in, using your hips, as shown in Figure 242. Reach with your right arm and get into the position shown in Figure 243, with your arm behind your opponent's neck. Grab your left biceps tightly with your right hand. Scoot your body slightly to the left for better leverage and squeeze, using your traps and back muscles. The pressure for the finish is almost the same as with the rear naked choke.

As with the leg triangle, the arm triangle choke will not work if your grip is too loose. Also it is very important that you move your body to the side. It is still possible to finish the choke without moving, but it is much more difficult.

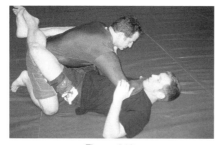

Figure 240.
Arm triangle, arm post on chest.

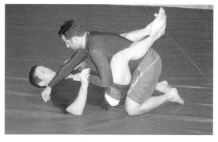

Figure 241.
Arm triangle, arm push.

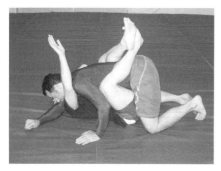

Figure 242.
Arm triangle, pull in and arm behind neck.

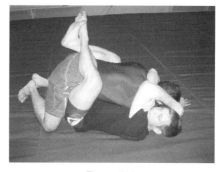

Figure 243.
Arm triangle, biceps grab.

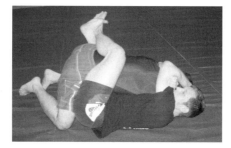

Figure 244.
Arm triangle, body scoot and squeeze.

Grappling Basics: A New Twist on Conditioning

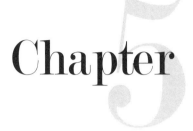

Exercises and Drills

Bodyweight exercises are staples of grappling training. Controlling and moving your own mass freely in all directions is a prerequisite for skill on the mat; thus, these types of exercises should be incorporated into all grapplers' training programs. There are many resources available for standard bodyweight training, such as Brad Johnson's *Bodyweight Exercises for Extraordinary Strength*; so we will confine our discussion to grappling-specific bodyweight drills, with which many non-grapplers may not be familiar. If you are training for grappling, these exercises have the dual benefit of being both skill and conditioning work. For non-grapplers, these exercises provide a novel and effective training stimulus that can spice up your normal routines.

Bodyweight Grappling Drills

Rope climbing

Rope climbing, although not exclusively a grappling exercise, is often used by grapplers to build grip and pulling power. Several different methods of climbing are available. The easiest technique is to keep the rope between your thighs and pinch it with your feet. Reach up, grip, and pull up your body with both hands; squeeze your thighs and feet to hold yourself in position while you reach up for a higher grip. A second, more difficult method is to simply climb hand-over-hand without any assistance from your lower body. Finally, for a real challenge, start seated on the floor and climb hand-over-hand while your body remains in the L-sit position.

Rope armbars

Stand next to a climbing rope and get a high grip with both hands. With a slight jumping motion, swing your lower body up until your feet are straight over your head, as shown in Figure 247. Drop back down and repeat. This exercise simulates an armbar and provides an excellent workout for your arms and core. To make the exercise more difficult, hang from the rope rather than stand on the floor between each rep.

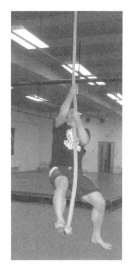

Figure 245.
Rope climbing,
hand-over-hand.

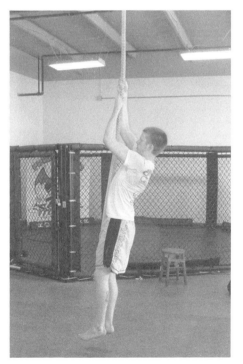

Figure 246.
Rope armbar, start.

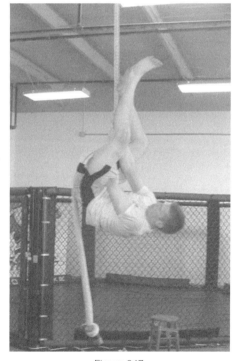

Figure 247.
Rope armbar, swing up.

Grappling Basics: A New Twist on Conditioning | **75**

Shrimping

Shrimping is a drill that teaches proper movement across the mat when you are on your back—a key component in many escape techniques. Start by lying flat on your back. Put your weight onto your left foot and right shoulder, turn to your right side, and push your butt out to the left, as shown in Figure 249. You are folding your body into the fetal position. Straighten out and repeat the same motion on the other side. You will move a short distance with each repetition. Gradually increase the movement speed as you become more proficient. Continue for the required number of repetitions, time interval, or distance.

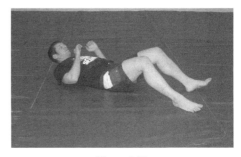

Figure 248.
Shrimping, start.

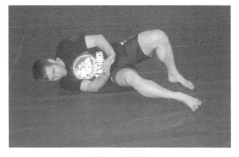

Figure 249.
Shrimping, turn and push to left.

Seated shrimping
Begin this drill by sitting down with your left leg bent and your right leg straight, as shown in Figure 251. Post your weight on your right hand and left foot and scoot your body backward. Switch to the other side, and post your weight on your right hand and left foot and scoot. Continue down the mat, switching sides each time.

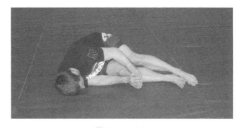

Figure 250.
Shrimping, fetal position.

Penetration step

The penetration step discussed in Chapter 2 (page 26) is a key component in the double-leg takedown. It is an excellent drill in its own right for developing lower-body strength and power. Start in a left-lead wrestling stance. Drive off your right foot and

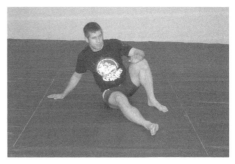

Figure 251.
Seated shrimping, start.

step forward with your left leg. Push onto the ball of your left foot and allow your knee to go forward and drop to the mat. Finish by sliding your right foot along the mat and return to standing. Repeat on the other side. Make sure that your elbows stay tight at your sides and that your chest faces forward throughout the exercise. Penetration steps can be rough on the tops of your feet as you slide along the mat, so wrestling shoes are recommended if you will be doing these for high repetitions or for a long distance.

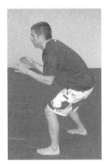
Figure 252. Penetration step, start.

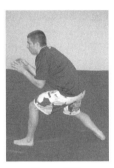
Figure 253. Penetration step, step forward.

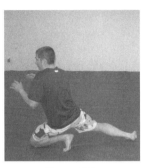
Figure 254. Penetration step, knee drop.

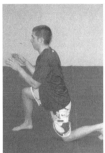
Figure 255. Penetration step, right foot slide.

Kimura sit-ups

Kimura sit-ups are a sit-up variant which simulates attacking the *kimura* arm lock from the guard. Start in a sit-up position, lying on your back with your knees bent. Post your left elbow on the mat and perform a twisting sit-up by bringing your right hand across your body to meet your left hand, as shown in Figure 257. Drop down and immediately repeat on the other side. Unlike with a traditional sit-up, you should attempt to utilize the momentum generated by the drop to explode into the next rep.

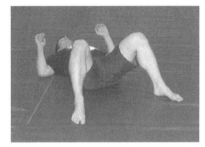
Figure 256. *Kimura* sit-ups, start.

These may also be performed with a partner to increase the realism. From a closed guard position, grab the opponent's right wrist with your left hand. Sit up and bring your right arm across his body and under his right arm until you grab your own left wrist with your right hand. Release and repeat on the other side.

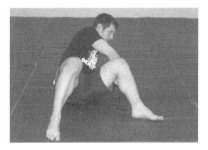
Figure 257. *Kimura* sit-ups, post and twist.

Rainbow

The rainbow exercise builds both rotational core strength and skill in escaping from the bottom position of certain pins. Lie flat on your back with your arms straight out to the sides. Bring your legs straight up into the air and cross your ankles, as shown in Figure 258. Lower your legs to one side and stop just short of touching the mat (Figure 259); reverse the direction and go to the other side. Try to keep your shoulders on the mat throughout the movement.

If you find this exercise too difficult, bend your knees to 90 degrees. As your strength builds, work into the straight-leg version. To make the exercise more difficult, move your legs in a complete circle rather than side to side. Start by lowering your legs to your left side; move them clockwise to the right, keeping your heels a short distance off the mat. Bring your legs back up to the center and repeat in the opposite direction.

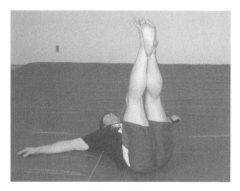

Figure 258.
Rainbow, start.

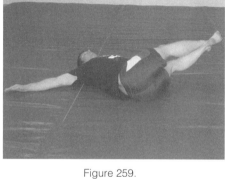

Figure 259.
Rainbow, legs to one side.

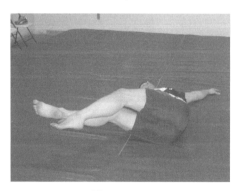

Figure 260.
Rainbow, legs to other side.

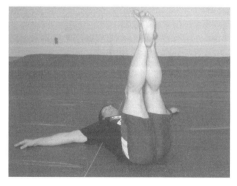

Figure 261.
Rainbow, back to center.

Hip-ups

Start in a seated position, with both feet straight out in front of you. Rock forward to touch your toes and then rock backward onto your shoulders, as shown in Figures 262 and 263. Point your toes and push your feet up toward the ceiling as you straighten your body. Lower your butt back to the mat, rock forward, and repeat for the required repetitions or time interval. Hip-ups condition your core and build dynamic flexibility.

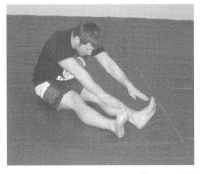
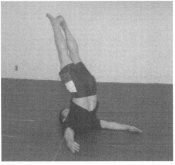

Figures 262 and 263.
Hip-ups, start and finish.

Solo sprawl drill

The sprawl is a fundamental defensive movement used against leg attack takedowns, such as single- or double-leg shots. Start in a basic wrestling stance, with your left leg forward. Drop your level quickly and kick your feet out behind you. Twist your left hip down so that your left leg is back farther than your right leg. You should land on the mat in the position shown in Figure 265. To soften the impact, make sure you practice this movement on a matted surface. You may also perform the solo sprawl using a heavy bag to further reduce shock and to simulate an attacking opponent. Put a heavy bag on the floor and stand over it so that when you sprawl, your hip drops on to the bag. The bag simulates your opponent and is softer than the floor.

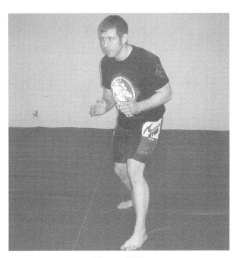

Figure 264.
Solo sprawl, basic wrestling stance.

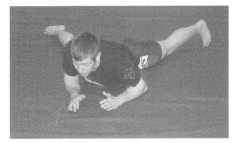

Figure 265.
Solo sprawl, landing position.

Grappling Basics: A New Twist on Conditioning | **79**

Body drag

The body drag conditions the arms, shoulders, and back. Lie flat on your stomach and reach out in front of you with both arms. Press your palms, forearms, and elbows into the mat and drag your body forward until your elbows are at your sides, as shown in Figure 267. Reach out again and repeat, dragging your body forward and pulling yourself all the way down the mat. Perform this drill for repetitions, distance, or time.

Bear and crab crawling

The bear crawl is performed by moving across the mat on all fours. Try to keep your hips down and move at a moderate, methodical pace rather than at a gallop. Work your arms and shoulders from different angles by crawling forward, backward, and sideways. For additional upper-body overload, incorporate push-ups at various intervals.

Crab crawling is done on all fours with the chest facing up. Your weight is distributed on your hands and feet and your butt stays off the mat. Do this exercise in all four directions.

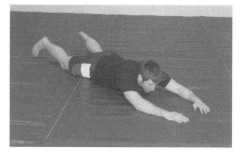

Figure 266.
Body drag, start.

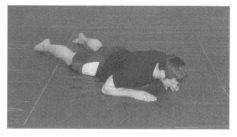

Figure 267.
Body drag, pull forward.

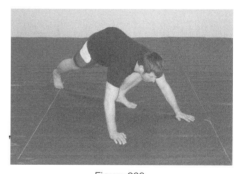

Figure 268.
Bear crawl.

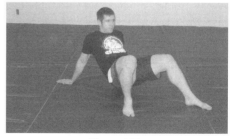

Figure 269.
Crab crawl.

Inchworm

Start from a standing position. Bend down, place both hands flat on the floor, and walk your body forward into a push-up position, as shown in Figure 271. Walk your feet up to meet your hands and repeat. This drill builds lower-body flexibility and endurance in the arms and shoulders. Repeat for a specified number of reps, or for distance or time. To increase the upper-body overload, add in a push-up when in the fully-extended position.

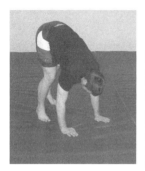
Figure 270.
Inchworm, start.

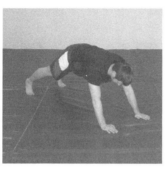
Figure 271.
Inchworm, walk hands out to push-up position.

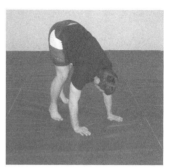
Figure 272.
Inchworm, walk feet in to finish.

Monkey walk

From a standing position, place your hands flat on the floor and walk out into a push-up position, as shown in Figure 273. Jump your feet up, landing next to your hands, as shown in Figure 274; repeat. Continue for reps, distance, or time. Add in a push-up in the extended position for extra upper-body work. The monkey walk is excellent training for your upper body and core.

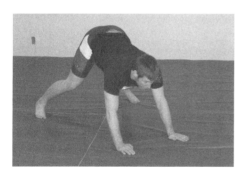
Figure 273.
Monkey walk, walk out to push-up position.

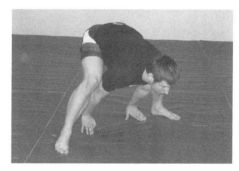
Figure 274.
Monkey walk, jump up.

Sit through

Begin this exercise in the push-up position. Raise your right arm off the mat, swing your left leg under you, twisting your body, and kick your right hand, as shown in Figure 276. During this motion, your body should twist so that your chest is facing to the left. Quickly bring your leg and hand back to their original position and repeat on the other side. Start slowly until you get the technique down, and gradually speed up. This endurance and shoulder stability exercise can be made even more demanding by performing a push-up after each switch.

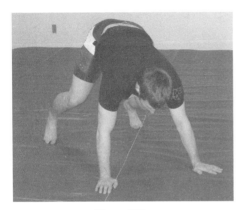

Figure 275.
Sit through, start.

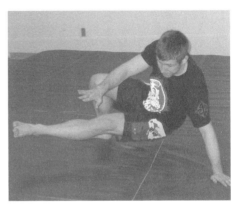

Figure 276.
Sit through, left leg swing and kick.

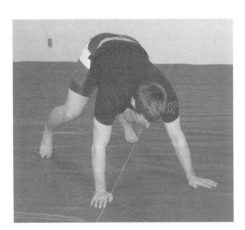

Figure 277.
Sit through, return to start.

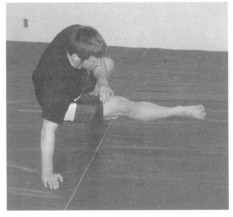

Figure 278.
Sit through, right leg swing and kick.

All fours spins

Start on all fours, with your chest facing the mat. Lift your right foot and left hand from the mat, and rotate your body so that your chest is facing upward and your right foot and left hand have switched places, as shown in Figure 281. Lift your right foot and left hand again and rotate so that your chest is once more facing the mat. Be sure that during the switch, your leg moves under your body. Start slowly to build technique and gradually increase the pace for a better conditioning workout. Do the drill for reps or time and be sure to work both directions equally. Practice switching directions fluidly or at a training partner's verbal command.

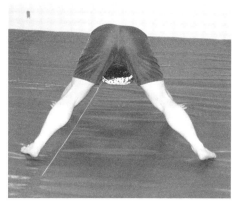

Figure 279.
All fours spin, start.

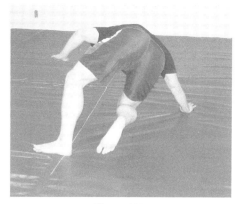

Figure 280.
All fours spin, lift and rotate.

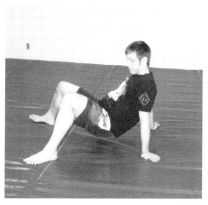

Figure 281.
All fours spin, finish.

Grappling Basics: A New Twist on Conditioning | **83**

Triangles

This exercise builds skill with the triangle choke from the guard and is an excellent abdominal and hip workout. Start flat on your back. Open your legs, rock back onto your shoulders, and swing to the left, making a figure four with your legs, as shown in Figure 283. Open your legs, swing your body to the right, and make a figure four with your legs on the opposite side. Repeat for the required number of reps or time interval.

Leg circling

Leg circling will develop your ability to use your legs when your opponent is in your guard, and it increases hip, leg, and abdominal endurance. Keep your lower legs loose and move them together in quick circles. Move your hips from side to side as you circle your legs. Perform this drill in both directions for reps or time.

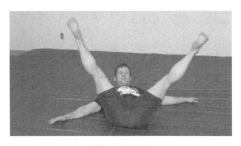

Figure 282.
Triangle, start.

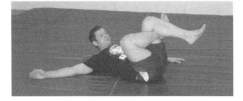

Figure 283.
Triangle, figure four, left side.

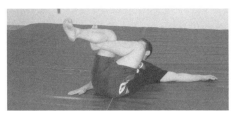

Figure 284.
Triangle, figure four, right side.

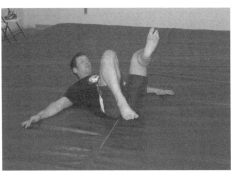
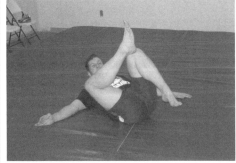

Figures 285 and 286.
Leg circling.

Legs over head

Sit on the mat with your feet straight out in front of you. Rock back and throw your feet over your right shoulder, as shown in Figure 288. Push off with the balls of your feet and rock back up to a seated position. Repeat on the other side. Be sure to move your head to the side just as in the backward roll so that you don't hurt your neck. Continue the exercise for the specified reps or time interval.

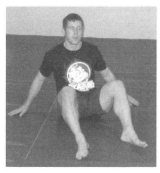

Figure 287.
Legs over head, start.

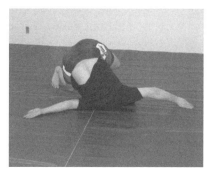

Figure 288.
Legs over head, right shoulder.

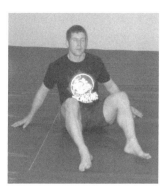

Figure 289.
Legs over head, return to start.

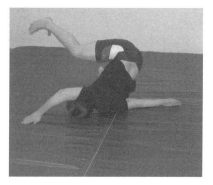

Figure 290.
Legs over head, left shoulder.

Wall walking

A drill for back and core strength and flexibility, the wall walk is used to teach wrestlers and other grapplers how to execute the lifting throws, such as the suplex. Start a few feet from a wall, facing away. Look up and bend backward until your hands reach the wall, as shown in Figure 292. Walk your body down until you end in a back bridge with your head on the mat, as shown in Figure 293. Reverse directions and walk back up the wall into a standing position. The fear of falling is natural and it takes some time to overcome it. Have a partner stand near to spot you if necessary, or only walk down a short distance at first. Walk closer to the mat as you develop more strength and technique.

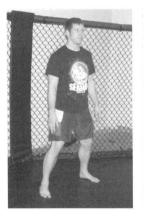
Figure 291.
Wall walking, start.

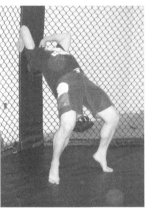
Figure 292.
Wall walking, backward bend.

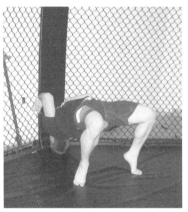
Figure 293.
Wall walking, bridge position.

Bridging (shoulder)

The shoulder bridge is a primary component of many ground escapes and a fundamental grappling movement. It builds strength and flexibility in the hips and core. Start the exercise by lying flat on your back with your knees bent at about 90 degrees. Press off your toes and drive your hips into the air, as shown in Figure 294. Drop your hips back to the mat and repeat. A more difficult version is the single-leg bridge, in which the same movement is done with one leg extended straight up.

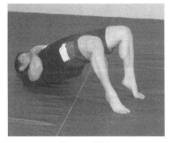
Figure 294.
Shoulder bridging.

The twisting bridge adds a core rotation component. Bridge up onto your right shoulder and reach across your body with your left arm. Drop back to the mat and repeat on the other side. Bridges may be performed for a set number of reps or continuously for time.

Bridging (neck)

Neck bridging is a basic exercise used by freestyle and Greco-Roman wrestlers to build skill in certain lifting throws, and to defend against having their shoulders pinned to the mat. Start flat on your back and press your hips up so that only your head, palms, and toes remain on the mat, as shown in Figure 295. As you become stronger and more flexible, increase the arch in your back by rolling farther onto the top of your head and bringing your feet closer to your head. From the bridge position, rock your weight back toward your head and forward toward your toes—this will help to build your strength. One up–down sequence is one rep.

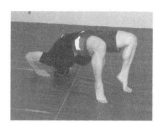

Figure 295.
Neck bridge.

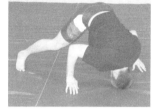

Figure 296.
Front neck bridge.

The front neck bridge is done facing the mat. Bring your hips off the mat so that only your head, palms, and balls of your feet remain on the mat, as shown in Figure 296. Rock forward and backward while in the top position. Both the front and back neck bridge may be done as an isometric hold for time or for a certain number of reps.

Standing guard pass drill

Have your partner lie flat on his back, with his feet at your hips; grab his ankles lightly with each hand. In one quick movement, toss his legs to the right and step your right foot close to his left hip, as shown in Figure 298. Step your left foot up to maintain balance. Move back to the start position and repeat the motion to the other side. This drill builds guard-passing skill and agility, and is a metabolic conditioner when performed for high repetitions or long durations.

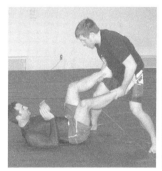
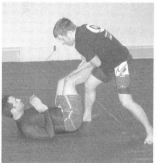
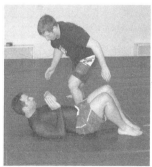

Figure 297.
Standing guard pass drill, ankle grab.

Figure 298.
Standing guard pass drill, leg toss.

Figure 299.
Standing guard pass drill, step to hip.

Grappling Basics: A New Twist on Conditioning

Chest-to-back spin drill

For the spin drill you will need a partner. Have your partner get on all fours and get on top of him with your chest on his back. Shift your weight onto your partner's upper back and keep only the balls of your feet in contact with the mat. Begin circling your partner's body, using your hands to help maintain your balance. Perform the required repetitions or time interval and be sure to do the same amount of work in both directions. Add a further reaction component by having your partner call out directional switches: when you hear the command, immediately begin moving in that direction.

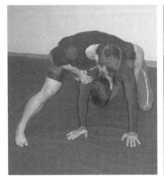
Figure 300.
Chest-to-back spin drill, start.

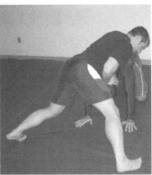
Figure 301.
Chest-to-back spin drill, spin.

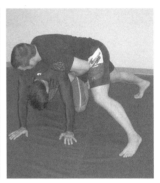
Figure 302.
Chest-to-back spin drill, finish.

Over and unders

The over and under drill is an anaerobic conditioner. Your partner stands facing you with his legs wider than shoulder-width apart. Squat down and shoot through his legs as quickly as possible. Immediately stand up, turn and place your hands on your partner's back, and vault over him. Once you land, turn and complete the next repetition as quickly as possible. Continue for the required reps or time interval.

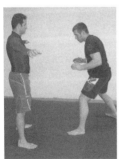
Figure 303.
Over and unders, face partner.

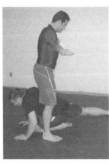
Figure 304.
Over and unders, squat and shoot.

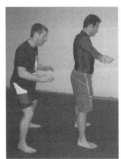
Figure 305.
Over and unders, turn.

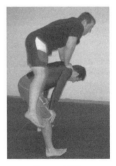
Figure 306.
Over and unders, vault.

Partner Resistance Training

Partner resistance training has been a key feature of grappling training since ancient times, and for good reason. If much of your sport involves lifting, moving around, or fighting against another person, it is difficult to find a more applicable training method than partner resistance. Unlike with barbells and dumbbells, human bodyweight is unevenly distributed, and finding an appropriate grip can be difficult. Partner resistance training is, then, skill training in a sense. In addition to building strength and muscle mass, you will develop technique and a "groove" for lifting your partner just as you did when you first began lifting free weights. The added factor of movement by the human weight presents challenges to core stability, balance, and grip. For grapplers, partner work translates to more effective technique on the mat. Non-grapplers can incorporate partner lifts as a new and unusual training stimulus that requires no equipment.

Ideally you and your partner will be close to the same weight and roughly equal in strength. In the case of a size or strength differential, modify the number of reps or duration. Some of these drills can also be performed with a sandbag or grappling dummy if your partner is too large or you work out alone. It may be prudent to spend some time learning how to fall and training on a matted surface in case you drop your partner.

Lifting

Leg press
Lie on your back and have your partner stand in front of you. Place your feet on his hips as he leans forward, as shown in Figure 307. Draw your knees toward your chest as far as possible and perform a leg press with his bodyweight. For most experienced lifters and grapplers, this drill is not too difficult and thus is typically performed for high-rep sets or time intervals. To increase the overload, use one leg at a time. For the single-leg version, place your foot on your partner's stomach and have him stabilize it with both hands.

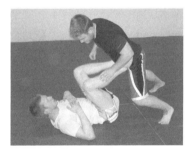

Figure 307.
Leg press, start.

Grappling Basics: A New Twist on Conditioning | 89

Leg press overhead

A more difficult variation of the leg press involves pressing your partner straight overhead. From the supine position, grab his wrists, and place your feet on his hips with your toes pointed slightly outward. Draw him in by bending your knees to your chest. Pull his wrists toward your head and press him straight up in the air. You may either return him to the mat after each rep or balance him overhead for the entire set. The key to keeping him balanced is to make sure that his head remains directly over your head during the set. Do not allow his weight to drift too far back or to the sides. If he comes too far forward and starts to fall, he should execute a forward roll to avoid injury.

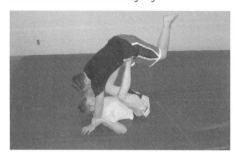

Figures 308.
Leg press overhead, wrist grab and feet on hips.

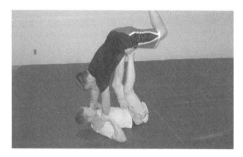

Figures 309.
Leg press overhead, press straight up.

Body-lock lift

Start a couple of feet away from your partner. Drop your level slightly, step in, and take a front, side, or rear body-lock on him. Lift your partner off the mat with an explosive drive from your hips and back, as shown in Figure 311. Drop him back down, and repeat. Make sure to grip around his waist rather than high up on his chest. Keep your head up and your back straight as if you were deadlifting. The head and leg grip variation shown in Figures 312 and 313 also works well for this drill.

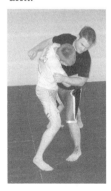
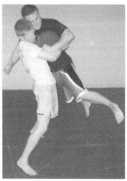
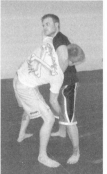
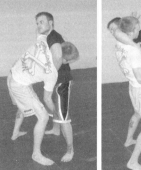

Figure 310.
Body-lock lift, drop and body lock.

Figure 311.
Body-lock lift, explosive lift.

Figures 312 and 313.
Body-lock lift, head and leg grip variation.

Double-leg lift
Practice your double-legs and build total body strength with the double-leg lift drill. Shoot in for a double-leg takedown (see pages 26–27) on your partner. Have your partner fall forward slightly to drape himself over your shoulder. Look up, step forward, and stand with your partner. Drop him back to the mat and repeat by shooting with the other leg. Do the same number of reps off both legs. For a more intense leg workout, hold your partner and perform a set of squats before setting him down.

Zercher lift
Have your partner sit down in the position shown in Figure 314. Squat down low and pick him up, with one hand under his lower back and the other in the crooks of his knees. Deadlift him off the ground, as shown in Figure 315, in a motion like the barbell Zercher lift. For added leg work, perform squats before returning him to the mat.

A variation is to catch your partner in this holding position as he jumps to you. Dip slightly and brace yourself for the landing. Once you have secured him, perform a set of squats, and then let him down.

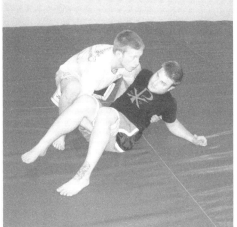 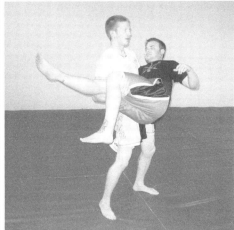

Figures 314 and 315.
Zercher lift.

Fireman's carry (standing and floor)

Squat down and lift your partner into the fireman's carry position, as shown in Figures 316 and 317. Performed for high reps or with a heavy partner, this hoisting movement alone can make an excellent workout. For added lower-body involvement, do a set of squats before returning your partner to the mat. The fireman's lift can also be done from a dropped-knee position. Start as shown in Figure 318: drop down to one knee, load your partner onto your shoulders, and stand up. Be sure to do an equal number of reps on each side.

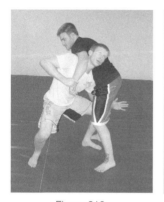
Figure 316.
Fireman's carry, squat set-up.

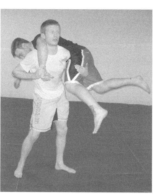
Figure 317.
Fireman's carry, stand.

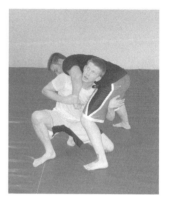
Figure 318.
Fireman's carry, dropped-knee set-up.

Guard lift

The guard lift develops skill and strength in guard passing. Begin in your partner's closed guard, as shown in Figure 319. Grab him under his shoulders with both arms and jump your feet forward into a deadlift position, as shown in Figure 320. Look up, arch your back, and stand (Figure 321). At the top, you can have your partner drop off you in order to avoid the eccentric motion, or you can lower him to the mat under control. Use caution when lowering someone heavy or training to extreme fatigue as you may accidentally slam your training partner and injure him.

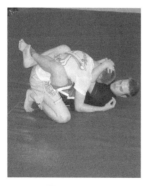
Figure 319.
Guard lift, start.

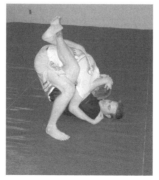
Figure 320.
Guard lift, deadlift position.

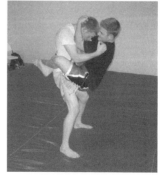
Figure 321.
Guard lift, lift and stand.

Stone lift

Have your training partner assume a "turtle" position. Reach down, bear hug his waist, and lift him by standing up, as shown in Figure 323. This exercise is similar to a round-back deadlift and is a common movement in freestyle and Greco wrestling. For variety and added stress on the core, start with your partner beside you rather than in front of you.

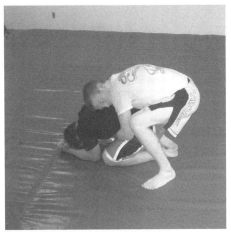

Figure 322.
Stone lift, start.

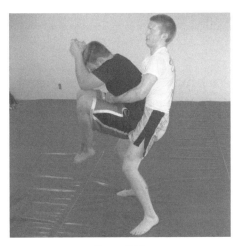

Figure 323.
Stone lift, stand and lift.

Partner deadlift

For this exercise, have your training partner lie down with a beach towel under his lower back. Stand over him, bend down, and get a grip on the ends of the towel. Perform a standard deadlift with your partner's bodyweight. If you have a *gi* top, have the down man wear it and lift him using a lapel grip. To assist you in this lift, have your partner remain as rigid as possible. Depending on your height, you may need to choke up on the towel or stand on two boxes to get an appropriate range of motion. In addition to strengthening your hips, legs, and lower back, grasping the towel places great stress on your grip.

Carry and drag

Carry from various hold positions

Carrying your training partner around the mat builds total body strength and is an excellent anaerobic conditioning exercise. There are several different grappling carrying positions—body-lock, fireman's carry, guard position, partner on back, Zercher, stone lift—each one placing stress on different areas of the upper body and core. Hoist your partner into position and perform carries for time, distance, or reps. Be sure that you have a firm grip, and use a matted or padded surface in case you drop him.

Wounded buddy drag

Have your training partner sit down with his legs straight out in front of him. Stand behind him, grip under his arms, and lift him so that only his heels or lower legs are on the mat, as shown in Figure 324. Drag him backward for the specified distance or time interval. When performing this movement on certain surfaces (such as a basketball court), a towel may be placed under his feet to help reduce friction.

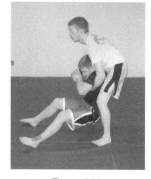

Figure 324.
Wounded buddy drag.

Pushing

Partner shove drill

The partner shove drill builds strength, power, and endurance in the upper body and teaches you how to use your entire body to drive your opponent back. It also provides a considerable anaerobic conditioning workout. Start facing your partner in the stance shown in Figure 325. Move in close and push him back with an explosive full-body drive, as shown in Figure 326. Move forward and repeat for the required number of reps, time interval, or distance. Make sure you lower your stance and drive with the legs as well as the arms for maximum power. Your partner should be in a strong stance as well, yielding just enough to allow full extension of your arms during the push. As a safety precaution, be sure that you are on a padded surface and that there is nothing behind your training partner that he might trip over or fall on.

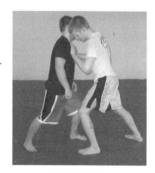

Figure 325.
Partner shove, start.

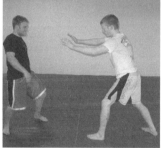

Hip bump and press

Begin this drill lying on your back with your partner mounted on you. Tuck your elbows close to your body and place your hands on your partner's hips.

Figure 326.
Partner shove, push back.

Lift your partner with an explosive drive from your hips combined with a bench press motion. Lock your elbows out at the top as you drop your hips back to the mat, as illustrated in Figure 329. Lower your partner and repeat. An alternate method for finishing this drill is to throw your partner to the side at the top of the lift and get back to your feet as quickly as possible. This builds strength and power while teaching a fundamental escape movement.

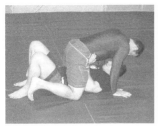
Figure 327.
Hip bump and press,
hands on hips.

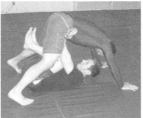
Figure 328.
Hip bump and press,
lift and drive.

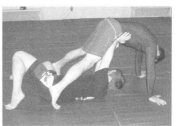
Figure 329.
Hip bump and press,
elbow lock and hip drop.

Partner push-up bench press

Lie flat on your back with your arms extended in a bench press lockout position. Your partner is in a push-up position on top of you with his hands on your hands, as shown in Figure 330. Execute a bench press; remain in the lockout position as your partner performs a push-up.

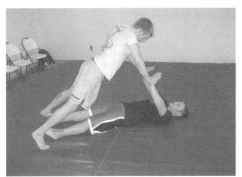
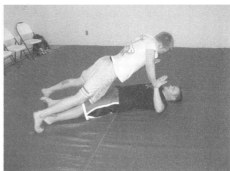

Figures 330 and 331.
Partner push-up bench press.

Resisted push-ups

Perform different push-up variations with your training partner providing resistance. Several different methods may be used. First, you can have your partner press down on your upper back, or if you are strong enough, sit on your shoulders. Another variation is to have your partner assume a push-up position on your back and do his own set while you perform yours, as shown in Figure 332. This is time-efficient and forces you to stabilize a moving load. A third method is to have your partner rest his feet on your shoulders or back and perform push-ups. This one also has a stabilization component.

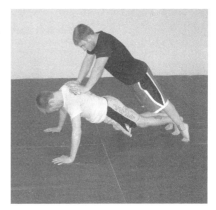
Figure 332.
Partner resisted push-ups.

Grappling Basics: A New Twist on Conditioning | **95**

Pulling

Bent-over row

This is a partner version of the standard bent-over row that places extra emphasis on the grip and provides a workout for both people. Have your partner lie flat on his back with his arms extended straight up. Stand over him, straddling his body at about stomach level. Reach down and grip your partner's forearms and have him grip your forearms as well, as shown in Figure 333. Row your partner's bodyweight up as if performing a barbell row. Your partner should keep his body as straight and rigid as possible during the exercise.

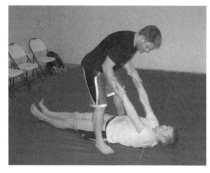

Figure 333.
Bent-over row, grip.

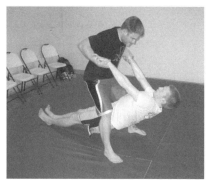

Figure 334.
Bent-over row, row partner.

Variations of this exercise can be done using a *gi* top. For the first variation have the down man wearing the *gi*. Rather than gripping his arms, grab the lapels of his top and row. You may also have the up man wearing the top. In this case, the up man bends over slightly farther and the down man executes a reclining pull-up by gripping the lapels.

Belt pulling

A belt (used in *gi* grappling sports), towel, or rope may be used for partner-resisted pulling exercises. Hold the belt in both hands with your arms fully extended while your partner holds the other end with his arms flexed. Pull the belt through the range of motion while your partner provides a moderate amount of resistance. He should adjust the resistance so that the exercise is difficult, but not impossible. Once you have completed your rep, reverse roles and provide resistance for your partner.

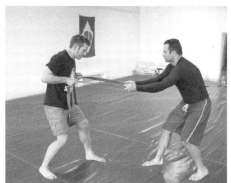

Figure 335.
Belt pulling, standing.

There are many variations of this drill to train all angles of the pull. The belt may be doubled over so that you have one end in each hand with your partner gripping the middle. The angle of the pull will depend on the relationship between you and your training partner. Figures 335 and 336 illustrate some of these variations.

Towel snaps

This exercise has been used in judo and grappling to improve grip, arm, and shoulder conditioning. Grasp the end of a thick beach towel and have your training partner do the same with the other end. As quickly and forcefully as possible, snap the towel up and down, as shown in Figure 337. Your partner does the same thing. Keep moving as fast as you can and as long as you can. Continue for a specified duration or perform this drill as a contest to see who can go the longest.

Gi pulls

Gi pulls are used by judo and jiu-jitsu players to develop a strong pull for throws. You will need a judo or jiu-jitsu *gi* top for this exercise. Your partner kneels in front of you, as shown in Figure 338. Grab his *gi* by both lapels. Step back with your left leg, dip slightly at the knees, and pull upward as powerfully as possible as if performing a barbell high pull. Your partner will end up on his feet, as shown in Figure 339, at the completion of the movement. Step back with the right leg and repeat. Your partner assists slightly by coming easily to his feet when you pull and adjusts the resistance so that you can complete the exercise properly. Be careful not to pull your partner's head into your face.

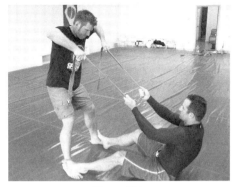

Figure 336.
Belt pulling, seated.

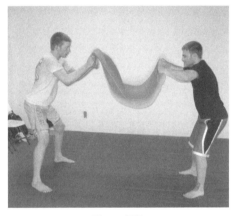

Figure 337.
Towel snaps.

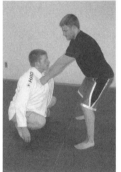 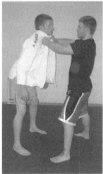

Figure 338.   Figure 339.
Gi pull, start.   *Gi* pull, finish.

Grappling Basics: A New Twist on Conditioning | **97**

Neck wrestling

This is a combative drill intended to improve your ability to maintain proper posture and body position against resistance. Face off with your training partner in a solid wrestling stance. Make sure your head is up and your back is straight. Your goal is to maintain your stance while your partner attempts to pull your head forward and sideways to knock you off balance. He may grab behind your head with one or both hands and push or pull you in any direction. His goal is to force your head forward so that you are looking at the mat or to snap you down so that you land on all fours (Figures 340 and 341). To prevent this, you must keep your neck tight and move your feet as he pulls or pushes so that your hips stay under you.

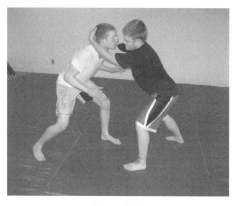

Figure 340.
Neck wrestling, head grab.

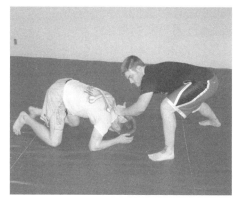

Figure 341.
Neck wrestling, snapdown.

Neck wrestling may be performed with only one partner attacking or with both partners attempting an offense. Perform this drill for timed rounds. A great metabolic conditioner, it will place enormous stress on your neck and upper-back muscles. It is recommended that you spend some time strengthening your neck with exercises such as bridges before attempting this drill.

Other partner drills

Single-leg balance drill

This drill is used to build balance for defending against single-leg takedowns. It is an excellent metabolic conditioner that builds tremendous leg endurance. Have your partner execute a single-leg entry—or grab—so that he begins the drill by holding your leg as shown in Figure 342. From here he attempts to take you down by moving you around to upset your balance. Repeat for a specified time interval; be sure to work both legs equally.

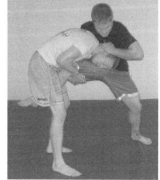

Figure 342.
Single-leg balance drill.

Change the intensity of the drill—how forcefully your partner moves you around—based on your skill level. It can be somewhat cooperative to fully competitive. Holding onto your partner will also make the drill easier.

Wheelbarrow
This is a classic partner exercise that provides a workout for both people simultaneously. Get into a push-up position and have your partner lift your legs off the floor. Walk forward, backward, or sideways. Keep your back tight so that your hips do not sag toward the floor. This drill is excellent for arm and shoulder endurance, and your partner will get some core and isometric upper-body work from holding you up. To make the exercise more difficult, add in push-ups every few feet, or move by hopping on your arms rather than walking. The most advanced version involves walking up stairs while in this position.

Guard sit-ups
Guard sit-ups build total-body strength with an emphasis on the core. Grab your partner's head and jump up into a standing guard position. Keep your legs locked tightly around his waist so that you don't slip off. Your partner should bend his knees and maintain as stable a posture as possible. Bend backward and perform a sit-up while maintaining guard. If you are strong enough, try to go all the way down until your head is near the floor, as shown in Figure 343.

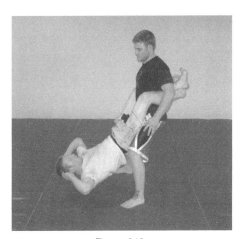
Figure 343.
Guard sit-ups, extension.

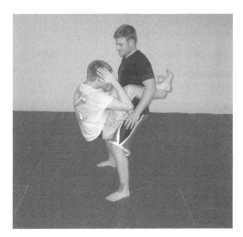
Figure 344.
Guard sit-ups, raise up.

Monkey climb

This is an advanced drill that develops strength in both partners simultaneously. Have your partner stand in a solid stance with his arms straight out at his sides. Jump onto his back and wrap your legs around him as shown in Figure 345. Without touching the floor, climb all the way around his body. Keep your legs clamped as tightly as you can to prevent sliding down. Monkey climbs work best when you and your partner are roughly the same size or if the climber is smaller. Do not attempt this drill if the person climbing is much larger.

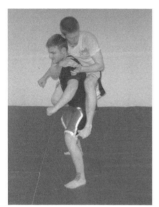 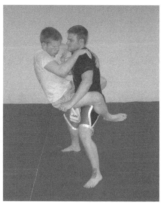 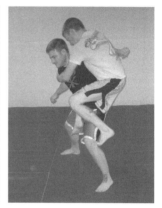

Figures 345–347.
Monkey climb around body.

Get-back-to-feet drill

This drill teaches you to defend against a standing opponent while you are on the ground. Start on the ground in the position shown in Figure 348, with your partner standing in front of you.

As your partner moves in a circle to your left, use your right foot and left hand to spin yourself in a circle to your left. If he switches directions and moves to the right, switch to the opposite position and begin spinning to the right. If your partner steps in close, rock back onto your shoulders and bring your knees to your chest to prevent him from getting on top of you, as shown in Figure 349. If he steps back a couple of steps, take the opportunity to stand up quickly, using the technique covered in Chapter 1 (page 18) and shown in Figure 350.

When learning the get-back-to-feet drill, have your partner move slowly. As your skill increases, your partner should speed up his movements. A more combative version involves your partner's attempting to get around your guard and prevent you from standing up by shoving you back to the mat as you try to stand.

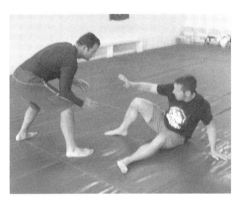
Figure 348.
Get-back-to-feet drill, spin to left.

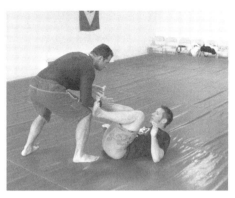
Figure 349.
Get-back-to-feet drill, knees to chest.

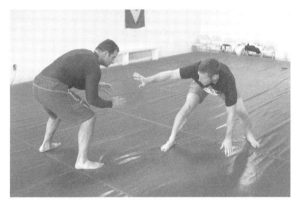
Figure 350.
Get-back-to-feet drill, stand up.

Grappling Basics: A New Twist on Conditioning | **101**

Chapter 6 — Workout and Program Design

Incorporating grappling drills can sometimes be a challenge to trainees who are used to setting up their workouts and programs based on body parts or muscle groups. While some of the exercises covered in this book may primarily work one area of the body, most are not easily classified. People new to grappling should begin with the movement drills and work sequentially through the book. Takedowns and clinch work require a proficiency in movement and balance, and submissions should not be attempted until one is proficient at the positions and escapes.

•Within each section, start with simple movements and progress to the more complex; you should also start at a slow speed and work more quickly as you gain proficiency in a movement.

•When working with a training partner, start with a cooperative method and work toward a competitive method once a base level of proficiency is developed.

Workout approaches

Perhaps the most comprehensive training method is to undertake a serious and long-term study of some grappling arts. Grappling has become more popular in recent years with the mainstream success of mixed martial arts competitions, such as the Ultimate Fighting Championship, Pride, and King of the Cage. As a result, wrestling, judo, Brazilian jiu-jitsu, and sambo schools have popped up in most areas of the U.S. Consider finding a school and devoting some time to learning grappling for its own sake. In addition to health and physical fitness, these arts are excellent for teaching self-defense, confidence, discipline, and mental toughness. Grappling emphasizes live training drills and sparring rather than pre-arranged sequences or *kata*. This focus means that fighting ability and competitive skill are developed more quickly compared to some traditional martial arts.

If there is no school nearby or if your budget is limited, much progress can be made with a motivated training partner and books or videos. Learn the basic techniques covered in this book and look into buying some of the many grappling DVDs now available. If you have Internet access, you will find many excellent video clips posted on different websites. Practice these techniques with your training partner(s) and add more people to your training group whenever possible.

Although long-term study of grappling will definitely take the guesswork out of program design, many people may not have the time, resources, or inclination to take up the art full-time. Those people should use one of the following approaches to training:

• **Short cycle:** Create a self-contained 2- to 4-week program based entirely around bodyweight, partner, and grappling drills. Practice is training, so focus extensively on technique to build skill and conditioning at the same time. Grappling training will provide an effective training stimulus without large external loads. This variation is particularly useful if you have just come off a longer cycle of heavy lifting and need to give your joints a break, or if you have been out of training and want to ease back into a program. If sparring and combative drills are emphasized, the short cycle can be extremely high-intensity and somewhat punishing on the body. Be sure that the exercises and drills you use fit your goals.

• **Dynamic warm-up or active recovery:** Current research has shown the need for flexibility and the superiority of a dynamic warm-up to static stretching prior to lifting. Many of the basic grappling movements, including falls, rolls, and mat mobility work, are effective warm-up drills. A key feature of most grappling exercises is its emphasis on the core, an area that needs special attention when warming up. A set of exercises lasting 5 to 10 minutes is ideal before any lifting session. On your off-days, the same exercises used for the warm-up can help speed recovery by flushing the sore areas with blood. Extend the warm-up to 10 to 20 minutes for an effective active recovery workout.

• **Integration method:** Choose one or more drills and insert them into your current workout routine in addition to, or instead of, other standard resistance or conditioning exercises. To determine where they best fit, use some common sense. Place squatting- or deadlifting-type movements into your lower-body workouts, pushing and pulling motions into your upper-body workouts, and full-body exercises anywhere you see fit.

Short Cycle Workouts

Two examples of the short cycle workout follow. The first is a combined bodyweight and grappling drill program that can be done solo, and the second can be used when you have a training partner.

Solo training – short cycle workout

Monday
- circuit A – x4 with 30–60 sec. rest between circuits
  - push-ups x25
  - back falls x15
  - triangles x 20
- circuit B – x4 with 30–60 sec. rest between circuits
  - pull-ups x10
  - side falls x20 (alternate sides each time)
  - hip bridges x30
- circuit C – x4 with 30–60 sec. rest between circuits
  - bodyweight squats x30
  - penetration step x10
  - rainbows x20

Wednesday
- circuit A – x4 with 30–60 sec. rest between circuits
  - walking lunges x30
  - shrimping x20
  - *kimura* sit-ups x20
- circuit B – x4 with 30–60 sec. rest between circuits
  - rope climb x3 (15–20 ft.)
  - sit throughs x20
  - legs over head x20
- circuit C – x4 with 30–60 sec. rest between circuits
  - bodyweight dips x15
  - leg circling x20/direction
  - all fours spin x10/direction

Solo training – short cycle workout (cont.)

Friday
- circuit A – x4 with 30–60 sec. rest between circuits
  - reclining pull-ups x15
  - forward rolls x15
  - hip-ups x25
- circuit B – x4 with 30–60 sec. rest between circuits
  - Hindu push-ups* x15
  - back rolls x15
  - rope armbars x8
- circuit C – x4 with 30–60 sec. rest between circuits
  - side lunges x30
  - seated shrimping x20
  - sprawls x15

* Hindu push-ups: Start in a push-up position with your rear in the air; descend while moving forward, just touching your chest to the floor. Finish in an arched-back position. Reverse the movement back to the starting position.

Partner training – short cycle workout

Monday
- weighted pull-ups 5 x 5 or 5–4–3–2–1
- pummeling 3 x 2 min; 30 sec. rests
- hip toss 5 x 10 on each side
  - do 10 throws in a row and rest as your partner goes
- shrimping 3 x 50 feet

Wednesday
- front squats 5 x 5 or 5–4–3–2–1
- partner body-lock and lift 5 x 10
- partner chest-to-back spin 5 x 10/direction
- knee tuck sit-ups 5 x 20

Friday
- weighted dips 5 x 5 or 5–4–3–2–1
- partner hip bump and press 5 x 15
- over and unders 5 x 10
- hanging leg raises 5 x 10

Dynamic Workouts

Repeat this circuit 2–3 times

- breakfalls   5 each to right, left, rear
- bodyweight squats   20
- bear crawl   10 yards
- seated shrimping   10 yards
- *kimura* sit-ups   20

Integration Workouts

These examples show how a few grappling exercises might be incorporated into your normal lifting routine over the course of a week. The lifting routine shown is a standard upper-body push, upper-body pull, and lower-body workout split.

Solo training – integration workout

Monday
- main lift – BB bent-over row (5x5 or 5–4–3–2–1 to top set)
- *gi* grip pull-ups 4 x 8–10
- body drag drill 5 x 25
- weighted incline sit-ups 4 x 10–15

Wednesday
- main lift – BB deadlift (5 x 3 or 5 x 1 to top set)
- lower-body and metabolic circuit x5, 60 sec. rest
  - single-leg hip bridge x10/leg
  - hip-ups x20
  - back fall and stand up x8/side
  - bodyweight squats x25
  - neck bridges x15

Friday
- main lift – BB overhead press (5x5 or 5–4–3–2–1 to top set)
- sit through with push-up 4 x 20

Solo training – integration workout (cont.)

Friday (cont.)
- Hindu push-ups* 4 x 15
- core circuit x3, no rest
  - *kimura* sit-ups x50
  - rainbows x30
  - leg circling x50/direction

* Hindu push-ups: Start in a push-up position with your rear in the air; descend while moving forward, just touching your chest to the floor. Finish in an arched-back position. Reverse the movement back to the starting position.

Partner training – integration workout

Monday
- main lift – bench press (5x5 or 5–4–3–2–1 to top set)
- partner shove
  - 4–5 sets of 50 feet (or continuously for 90 sec.)
  - alternate drill and rest while your partner goes
- bear crawl and push-up
  - crawl forward 50 feet, 5 push-ups, crawl backward 50 feet, 5 push-ups
  - do 4–5 sets; alternate work/rest with your partner
- abs/metabolic circuit x3, no rest between sets
  - weighted sit-ups x15
  - side-to-side triangle drill x20
  - burpees x10
  - back fall and stand up x10 (alternate sides each time)

Wednesday
- main lift – power cleans (5x5 or 5–4–3–2–1 to top set)
- partner bent-over rows
  - do 4–5 sets of 10–20 reps (or continuously for 90 sec.)
  - alternate drill and rest while your partner goes
- rope climb
  - 5 trips up a 15–20-ft. rope
  - alternate drill and rest while your partner goes
- partner guard sit-ups
  - do 4 sets of 5–10
  - alternate drill and rest while your partner goes

Grappling Basics: A New Twist on Conditioning | **107**

Partner training – integration workout (cont.)

Wednesday (cont.)
- metabolic work
  - neck wrestling 2 x 2 min. rounds, 30–60 sec. rest
  - sumo wrestling 2 x 2 min. rounds, 30–60 sec. rest

Friday
- main lift – back squats (5x5 or 5–4–3–2–1 to top set)
- partner stone lift
  - do 4–5 sets of 5–10 (or continuously for 90 sec.)
  - alternate drill and rest while your partner goes
- partner fireman's carry
  - lift your partner onto one shoulder and carry him 50 feet, put him down, switch shoulders, and repeat
  - do 4–5 sets (or continuously for 90 sec.)
  - alternate drill and rest while your partner goes
- abs/metabolic circuit x3
  - V-ups x15
  - forward rolls x20
  - Russian twist x20
  - penetration step shot x20

Combative Drilling and Conditioning

While there is a great deal of benefit in training competitively with your partner(s), a word of caution is in order: competitive drilling is extremely high-intensity, and the harder you go at it, the more likely you are to accumulate bumps, bruises, and strains. Getting banged-up in itself is no reason to avoid such training. However, if you are incorporating grappling work as a rest from heavy lifting, it is advisable to focus on the cooperative work. Just as with lifting, do not let your enthusiasm and intensity overstep the bounds of your skill. Technique must always come before resistance and competition. Always keep this in mind so that you can enjoy safe, productive training.

Grappling Basics: A New Twist on Conditioning | **109**

Index

A

Achilles lock 68-69
ankle pick 32-33
arm lock (see also armbars) 39-40, 55, 64, 77
arm triangle 72
armbars (arm locks) 64-68, 75
 cross armbar 65
 guard armbar 66
 bent arm lock (*kimura*) 67-68
 kimura 67, 77

B

back fall 11, 13, 104, 106-107
back mount 38-39, 52-53, 70
back mount escapes 52-53
backward trip 32
body-lock 21, 23, 35-36, 90, 93
body-lock and trip 35-36
bodyweight drills (see drills, bodyweight)
bottom game defense 40-41
breakfalls 11
bridge 41, 43, 45, 47-50, 86-87, 104, 106
 shoulder (hip) 86, 104
 neck 87, 106
bridge and roll 48, 50
Burns, Martin "Farmer" 3
cartwheels and roundoffs 16-17
chokes 38-40, 52-53, 64, 70-72
 rear naked choke 70, 72
 triangle choke 61, 70-72, 84
 arm triangle 72

C

clinch work (tie-ups) 4, 7, 20-25, 102
 wrist control 20-21
 hand fighting 21-22
 head and wrist tie-up 22
 over-and-under position 23
 front body lock 23
 pummeling 23-24, 35, 105
 head and elbow 24, 33
 two-on-one (Russian) 25
crawls 17-18, 80, 106-107
 bear crawl 18, 80, 106-107
 crab crawl 18, 80
cross side 38-39, 46, 50, 53-54, 58, 60-62, 68
cross side escapes 47-49
 shrimp out 47-48
 bridge and roll 48
 belly down 48-49

D

deadlift 91-93, 103, 106
double-leg takedown (see takedowns, double-leg)
double underhook 62
drills 4, 74-101, 103
 solo (see drills, bodyweight) 74-87
 partner (see drills, partner) 87-88
 partner resistance training (see drills, partner resistance) 89-101

D (cont.)
drills, bodyweight 74-87
 rope climbing 74-75, 104, 107
 rope armbars 75, 105
 shrimping 76, 104-106
 penetration step 76-77, 104, 108
 kimura sit-ups 77, 104, 106-107
 rainbow 78, 104, 107
 hip-ups 79, 105-106
 solo sprawl drill 79, 105
 body drag 80, 106
 bear and crab crawl 80, 106-107
 inchworm 81
 monkey walk 81
 sit through 82, 104, 106
 all fours spins 83, 104
 triangles 84, 104
 leg circling 84, 104, 107
 legs over head 85, 104
 wall walking 86
 bridging, shoulder 86, 106
 bridging, neck 87, 106
drills, partner 87-88
 standing guard pass drill 87
 chest-to-back spin drill 88, 105
 over and unders 88, 105
drills, partner resistance training 89-101
 lifting 89
  leg press 89
  leg press overhead 90
  body-lock lift 90, 93, 105
  double-leg lift 91
  Zercher lift 91, 93
  fireman's carry 92-93, 108
  guard lift 92-93
  stone lift 93, 108
  partner deadlift 93
 carry and drag 93
  carry in various positions 93
  wounded buddy drag 94
 pushing 94-95, 103
  partner shove drill 94, 107
  hip bump and press 94-95, 105
  partner push-up bench press 95
  resisted push-ups 95
 pulling 96-98, 103
  bent-over row 96, 107
  belt pulling 96-97
  towel snaps 97
  gi pulls 97
  neck wrestling 98, 107
 other 98-101
  single-leg balance drill 98-99
  wheelbarrow 99
  guard sit-ups 99, 107
  monkey climb 100
  get-back-to-feet drill 100-101
drive through 27-28

F

falling 11
    back fall 11-13, 104, 106-107
    side fall 11, 104
    front fall 12
    spin-out 12-13, 48
flare 31
footwork 4, 6, 8-9
    linear 8
    lateral 9
    circling 9, 29-30, 32, 88
freestyle 2, 12, 87, 93
front body-lock 23
front fall 12

G

gi 70, 93, 96-97, 106
Gilgamesh, Epic of 2
glima 2
Gotch, Frank 3
Greco-Roman 2, 12, 87, 93
grip, overhand 21
grip, underhand 21
ground positions 38-62
    mount 38-39, 41-43, 53-54, 56-58, 65, 94
    cross side 38-39, 46, 50, 53-54, 58, 60-62, 68
    scarf hold 33, 38-39, 49-50
    back mount 38-39, 52-53, 70
    guard 38-40, 43-45, 47, 52-60, 66-68, 70, 72, 77, 84, 87, 92-93, 100-101
guard 38-40, 43-45, 47, 52-60, 66-68, 70, 72, 77, 84, 87, 92-93, 100-101
    closed guard 44, 54, 59, 77, 92
    open guard 54
    bottom position 54-55
    guard sweeps 56-57
    guard passing 38, 54, 58-62, 87, 92
guard passing 38, 54, 58-62, 87, 92
    breaking the guard, guard break 59-60
    leg throw 60
    single underhook 61-62
    double underhook 62

H

Hackenschmidt, George 3
hand fighting 21-22
head and wrist tie-up 22, 32
head and elbow tie-up   24, 33
head lock 55
hip toss 33-34, 105

J

jiu-jitsu (Brazilian) 2, 11-12, 38, 52, 97, 102
joint locks 38, 64-69
    armbar 64-68
    leg locks 64, 68-69
judo 2, 11-12, 38, 52, 64, 70, 97, 102

K

kimura (see also armbar, *kimura*) 67, 77

L

leg lock 64, 68-69
    Achilles lock 68-69
leg throw 60
leg triangle 72
Leiderman, Earle 3
level change 10
    sprawling 10, 28, 79
    standing up 18, 101, 106

M

mount 38-39, 41-43, 53-54, 56-58, 65, 94
    high mount 41-43
    low mount 41, 43
mount escapes 43-45
    trap and roll 43
    shrimp out 44
    hip bump 45
movement 4, 6, 10, 76, 89

O

over-and-under position 23

P

pain compliance 64
panic 40-41
pankration 2
penetration step (shot) 10, 26-28, 32-33, 76-77, 104, 108
physical culture 3-4
pins 4, 38-62, 68, 78, 87
positioning (see ground positions)
posture 58
pull-ups 96, 104-105
pummeling 23-24, 35, 105
push-ups 80-82, 95, 100, 104-107
putting in hooks 52

R

rear naked choke 70, 72
rolling & tumbling 13, 103
    forward somersault roll 14, 105, 108
    backward somersault roll 14, 105
    forward shoulder roll 15
    backward shoulder roll 16
    cartwheels & roundoffs 16-17
run the pipe 30
Russian (see two-on-one)

S

sambo 2, 12, 38, 64, 102
Saxon, Arthur 3
scarf hold 33, 38-39, 49-50
scarf hold escapes 50-51
    bridge and roll 50
    twist out 51
self defense 64, 102
shot (see penetration step)
shoulder roll, backward 16
shoulder roll, forward 15
shrimp out 44, 47-48
shrimping 44, 76, 104-106
side fall 11, 104
single underhook 61
single-leg takedown (see takedowns, single-leg)

Grappling Basics: A New Twist on Conditioning | **111**

S (cont.)

sit-ups 77, 100, 104-107
snap-down 7
somersault roll, backward 14, 105
somersault roll, forward 14, 105, 108
space 41
specialization 3
spin-out 12, 48-49
sprawling 10, 28, 79, 105
squats 12-14, 16, 91-92, 103-106, 108
stances 4, 6-8, 79
    square 7, 9
    staggered 6-10, 29
stand-up grappling 4, 20
standing up 18, 101, 106
step behind trip 28
    crossover step 9
submission 2, 4, 12, 38-40, 43, 52, 54-55, 58-59, 64-72,
      102
    joint locks 38, 40, 64-69
    chokes 40, 64, 70-72
    pain compliance 64
suplex 86
sweeps 54-58
    scissors sweep 56
    sit-up sweep 57
swimming 23-24, 35, 41, 61-62
Swiss ball 40

T

takedowns 4, 7, 10-11, 13, 20-22, 24-36, 60, 102
    penetration step (shot) 10, 26-28, 32-33, 76-77,
        104, 108
    double-leg takedown 7, 26-29, 76-77, 79, 91
        drive through 27
        step behind trip 28
        turn the corner 28
    single-leg takedown 7, 26, 29-33, 79, 98
        run the pipe 30
        flare 31
        backward trip 32
        ankle pick 32-33
    hip toss 33-34
    body-lock and trip 35-36
tie-ups (see clinch work)
top game pressure 40
training programs 104-108
triangle choke 61, 70-72, 84
tumbling 13
turn the corner 28-29
turtling 52
two-on-one (Russian) 25
workouts 104-108
wrestling 2, 38, 52, 64, 86, 102
    sumo wrestling 107
wrist control 20-21
    overhand grip 21
    underhand grip 21